AGELESS SPINE, LASTING HEALTH

The Open Secret to Pain-Free Living and Comfortable Aging

Kathleen Porter

AGELESS SPINE, LASTING HEALTH:
THE OPEN SECRET TO PAIN-FREE LIVING AND COMFORTABLE AGING
PUBLISHED BY SYNERGY BOOKS
2100 Kramer Lane, Suite 300
Austin, Texas 78758

For more information about our books, please write to us, call 512.478.2028, or visit our website at www.bookpros.com.

Library of Congress Control Number: 2006923896

ISBN-10: 1-933538-40-6
ISBN-13: 978-1-933538-40-2

Publisher's Cataloging-in-Publication available upon request.

For Meredith, Kendra and Evan
Treasures of the heart

CONTENTS

ACKNOWLEDGMENTS

To say that I have struggled to land on my feet is an understatement. Luckily, I've had lots of help. I could fill the pages of another whole book with words of everlasting gratitude to the many people who have given me so much encouragement and support. Having this opportunity to acknowledge these people turns out to be the most gratifying detail of this entire project.

It is said that we are all students and teachers to each other. Nowhere has this been more clearly demonstrated than in the role reversal I have enjoyed in my ongoing association with Ho Sheng Chih, Hettie Scofield, Marianne Kuipers-Tilanus, Sandra Pickard, Phyllis Aguiar, Donna Perkins, Jan Cooper, Milo Jarvis, Sawami Mitamura and Linda Kennedy. Not only have these adventurous ones hung in there through the writing of and all the changes required for this book, they have also willingly ventured inside their own skins and shared their inner landscapes, so that we could all learn from each other. Out of this, we have also built friendships. I thank you all!

Other teachers have influenced me in important ways. No one is more responsible for this book than Jean Couch, mentor and friend, who held open the door and pointed the way, always with great generosity of spirit. Norman Skinner helped me put my boots on, among other things. Bruce Fertman long ago turned on a light and ignited a curiosity for what might be sensed and discovered. Jon Kabat-Zinn first introduced me to the organic healing power of silence. Kaila Kukla took me by the hand and led me along on whole new adventures. Carter Beckett taught me what is possible through compassionate Rolfing hands. Judith Aston brought ground-reaction force to life for me. Kamala Masters inspired me with gentle quietude. Sayadaw U Pandita kindly and resolutely pushed me to the edge. Maria Jaramillo showed how giving and receiving are the same. Rebecca Lux and Jeffrey Dann shared a wealth of information with me. I have learned much from the writings of a multitude of others, far too many to list here. I most especially appreciate the influence of J. Krishnamurti, a beacon to me for nearly 30 years, who helped me understand that truth is not a destination we can ever hope to reach but something to be discovered anew in each moment.

It is my good fortune to be the beneficiary of profoundly loving and sustaining friendships, without which I would surely have disintegrated long ago. Thea Beckett is a true sister of the heart and has nourished me with her goodwill and rich sense of humor for about as far back as I am able to remember. Her sustained enthusiasm for this project kept me going, and her keen insights kept me on track. Kathryn Grout is a stalwart and loving friend whose constant support and keen interest in these ideas has helped me in unbounded ways for many years. Anne Kokubun is my cherished buddy. Sally Mermel continues to be the glue, and so much more. Patricia Salmon is unendingly generous with her friendship and encouragement. Dianne Horwitz gives and shares so much with me, including a poodle named Slick and an adoptive family. Wendell Ing graces my life and everyone else's with openhearted acceptance and contagious laughter. Cindy Kusinski's good will is an ongoing blessing. Jan Cooper inspires me with her sincerity and instincts for goodness. Wendy Miyamoto materialized like a loving angel (she is one!) and single-handedly set the stage for wonderful things to come.

Throughout the years, Elaine Lee, Cindy Berry (along with Emma and Autumn), Patti Chikasuye, Linda Haynes, Ira Ono, Kenneth Lahti, Kathleen Golden, Peter Golden, Russell Kokubun, Cynee Wenner and Lorna Jeyte have given far, far more than I will ever know how to return. I thank Meredith Tedards, Daralyn Higgins, Monjuri Clarry, Moira Stratton, Suzanna Valerie, JoAnn Pobocik, Jeffrey Mermel, Cathy O'Reilly, Marilyn Nicholson, Kaila Kukla, Andre Kukla, Eva Lee, Chiu Leong, Pam Barton, Colleen Ziroli, Peter Ziroli, Terri Perreira, Sharon Mols, Barbara Heintz, Virginia Tench, Yumiko Kohama, Mary Goodrich, Lisa Louise Adams, Suzanna Saxton, Jon Beers, Marilyn Eto and Steve Fleisher for their enduring friendship. Added together, the blessings that have come my way through these openhearted friends encompass hundreds of years! I am joyfully indebted to my sweet sister friends Catherine Killam, Beth Stout, Emma (Flambe) McAlexander, Sharon Moraes, Sally (yet again!) Georgia Bannon, Janet Hara, Patty Bourke, Tricia Tierney and Debra Serrao—not to mention the center of our cyclone, Elaine Willis—for riotous good times and the part each has played in helping to birth me out of one life and into another. The resurrected Chevy Chase gang—Diane Parfitt, Nancy Morgan, Barb Isham, and Dotsy Smith—has delivered mountains of fun and tender reflections.

Weston Willard jumped into action more than once to lend his expertise, along with much good cheer, just when I needed it. Maile Kjargaard revealed to me what unconditional generosity looks like, and Trish and Russ Ellis demonstrated through their unrelenting dedication what living by principles of Attitudinal Healing looks like. My AH cohort facilitators—Barbara Green, Paula Thomas, Robert Searight, Fran Wiebenga, Marga Stammen, Jan Cooper and Marianne Kuipers-Tilanus—all practice (without preaching) unconditional love and acceptance. I thank Susan McCutcheon for opening her heart and her home to "the boys" and Greg Brenner for opening my eyes to many valuable things, both large and small. I benefited greatly from happy times spent with Gay Barfield. Da Gloors—Terrin, LeAna, Amira and Isaac—embody the best of what neighbors can be, and a neighborly thank you also goes to Joanne Kissler for her steady good vibes. Thank you Lynette Kanuha for your cheery presence and to Ann Fukuhara for helping to pull things together, yet again. *Muito obrigado* to Ana Rita Naciemento, Luis Santos and Dalia Santos for opening your loving hearts so wide to a traveling stranger. I thank Cathy Montvel-Cohen for staying until the very end, Susan O'Neill for living up to the fact she was voted friendliest person in her high school and Bing Summoto for being such a role model at ninety-two.

I humbly thank U Hla Myint, U Khin Hlaing, Sanh Nguyen and Du Tran for so graciously including me in the adventure of a lifetime and Daw Than Myint for helping to make it happen. Rinku Barua offered comforting friendship, and Ma Kamala brightened the darkness with the warmth of her smile. I wish to thank Sayadaw U Sasana for his constant words of encouragement and remarkable patience. I also owe a debt of gratitude to Putu Merta, Mr. Tho and Nyoman Puja, who understood what I was looking for and helped me find it.

A most appreciative thank you to Leah Morton, M.D., Christiane Northrup, M.D. and Ingrid Bacci, Ph.D. for generous words of encouragement and keen interest in these ideas. *Mahalo,* also, to Steve Bennett at Authorbytes.com for instant enthusiasm and his many obvious talents. Elsewhere in Cambridge, Carolyn Jenks has been cheering this on from the sidelines. I thank Jim Kennedy for holding my feet to the fire in a most friendly way.

A giant thank you to everyone at BookPros and Synergy Books for being most helpful and professional in lending their expertise, as well as being unendingly patient with me.

Thank you D'Arcy Nicola, and Jean Farmwald of the Balance Center along with Marilyn Basham and Mike Couch for being so welcoming—again and again. *Mahalo nui loa* to Sara Simmons and baby Kirra who so cheerfully joined in—just in the nick of time—and likewise to Camille and Carter Scofield for your help, too. Thank you to Cara Uyetake for such competent assistance.

I thank my late parents, Paul and Hilda Porter from the bottom of my heart for the gift of love that lives on and grows sweeter each day. I appreciate the love and support I receive from my brothers Dan, Jack and Ken Porter and their wonderful partners in life—Marianne Porter, Lisa Fuller and Debbie Porter—along with their beautiful, and expanding, families. I thank Janet Porter for many things, not the least of which is her part in bringing Kristin and Amy Porter into my life—and now Jack Nguyen, too. I thank my indomitable Aunt Peggy Kopmann for being such an inspiration to me and also Tobi Anderson and dear Al (whom we all miss) for good cheer and lively commentary over the years. Thanks to Barbara Hindley and Chuck Eisenhardt for the simple fact that just thinking of these kindred spirits brightens my day. I thank Lily and Wilfred Ing, now gone from us, for a list of kindnesses too long to recount, and Georgette and Michael Taylor, who so naturally carry on the family tradition of generosity.

And finally, with words that are inadequate to express my love and gratitude, I thank my children—Meredith, Kendra and Evan Ing. Each graces my life with the very best that life has to offer and teaches me by unique and shining example that the essence of our being is Love.

FOREWORD

Here's a quick start to understanding this whole book. The next time you lie down, lie on one side and take your free arm straight up into the air. Take a moment or two, and find the place where your arm is weightless. Notice how there are no tensions in the muscles and the joints have no stresses. If you close your eyes, you may feel that your arm has become invisible. When you find the place where gravity holds your arm, you may feel delighted at how easy this is to achieve and slightly euphoric from relief.

This is what it feels like to be in the NATURAL ALIGNMENT that Kathleen Porter describes in this book. It is possible for your whole body to be upright and to be internally supported in such a way that you feel weightless (at any weight!), where your muscles have no tension and your joints are fluid because they align as they are designed to. This book is the beginning of you having the info and the know-how to regain this natural state.

Not that it's going to be easy. Both Kathleen and I can tell you personal stories of how the information here rang true instantly, but giving up deep-seated beliefs and ingrained physical habits from years of out-of-aligned practice was maddening. However, you should be forewarned, once you comprehend the information in this book, it is hard to settle for less. Once you see what TRUE FITNESS is, it's hard to return to holding, lifting, tucking and tightening. You are embarking on a whole new mental, physical, spiritual journey that is going to amaze and delight you.

First in this book comes the very eloquent and thorough explanations of what NATURAL ALIGNMENT is, accompanied by the illuminating and inspiring photos of people from all around the world who never lost their NATURAL ALIGNMENT. Next, the chapters of exploration prepare the way for implementing the specific directions in the last section on what to do to feel weightless from moment to moment.

In the beginning, you follow guidelines. In time, you float.

Noelle Perez of the Institute D'Aplomb in Paris, France, pioneered the impetus for this work. Since 1959, she has been scrutinizing and describing the difference between people who have natural alignment and those who don't. From decades of empirical observations, the most basic tool of science, we are role-modeling the world's most successful postures, the world's most successful movement patterns.

Never before in the world of fitness has there been such a readable, groundbreaking, seminal book. Because you live in a human body and you were in natural alignment as a young child, a piece of your consciousness will recognize —you will intuitively re-know—how to optimize your relationship with gravity that will set you free in so many ways. Kathleen Porter, through this revolutionary book, is about to rock your world!

Jean Couch

Founder, The Balance Center

AUTHOR'S NOTE

In addition to addressing natural structural alignment, this book also touches on other themes. It is one part anthropology, one part physical therapy, one part travelogue, another part—a very big part, I hope—a plea for research into the health implications related to skeletal alignment.

Except to say that many of the photographs were taken in Myanmar (formerly Burma), Thailand, Vietnam, Indonesia, Portugal and England as well as in the United States, I have chosen to leave out details about the people, places and circumstances viewed in many of these photographs. One reason for this is to maintain strict focus on the central message of the book—the importance of natural spinal alignment of the human species, of which each of us is a part, no matter where in the world we happen to be. The greatest differences among peoples of the world are cultural, geographic, economic and religious. While far beyond the scope of this book, these differences cannot go unacknowledged. It is easy to romanticize the lives of women who can easily carry heavy loads on their heads while disregarding the often-difficult and unfair conditions in which so many people in the world are forced to live and work, frequently caused by such things as the long-term consequences of colonialism and exploitative economic practices.

This point touches on the fact that whenever photographs of unknown people are included in any book or magazine, it raises certain ethical questions that relate to issues of voyeurism and exploitation, no matter how we might try to justify our intentions. While some of the people who were photographed for this book quite willingly gave their permission, others did not have an opportunity to make that choice. In some cases, their images were "taken" without their knowledge. It is tempting for me to say I was justified in doing this because others will be helped by the examples revealed in the photographs.

I hope it is true that many people will be helped—indeed that is my motivation for writing this book—but I am not thoroughly convinced that this ends-justifies-the-means reasoning is acceptable. I wish to extend my personal gratitude to all the people whose images I have gathered here. I encourage anyone reading this to see the people inside these photographs rather than only seeing them as examples. I take full responsibility for the choices I have made here and sincerely hope that I have caused no harm.

American culture is difficult to define; we are such a diverse and multi-ethnic collection of people. Some Americans, because of their heritage or certain childhood influences, are less likely to be susceptible to conditioned beliefs and characteristics of the "dominant" culture, such as tucking their butts or sucking in their bellies. By dominant culture I mean the one that is almost single-mindedly promoted by mainstream media through television, magazines and movies as well as a steady bombardment of other messages we absorb in countless ways every day. This dominant culture sets the standard and spells out what is attractive, healthy, fit and acceptable while establishing deeply embedded beliefs in the psyches of many people in America. Generally, these "rules," though unconsciously mandated, are a departure from what is natural and healthy. An example of this is that "women, in order to be attractive, should have flat bellies."

That said, the words *we, our* and *us* are sometimes used in this book to refer to those who tend to be unconsciously conditioned and influenced by these mainstream messages. I put myself and almost everyone else in this country in that category. In other cases, *we* is used to refer to everyone's membership in the global human melting pot. Hoping that I have succeeded in making these distinctions clear, I leave it to the reader to determine how the use of "we" is intended in the context of any given passage.

One last note. A commonly held belief is the notion that less labor and greater wealth leads to a better life. Some people see physical labor as demeaning, as delegating them to a lower place on the status scale. After all, you don't need an advanced degree to dig a trench or build a rock wall. What is often overlooked is that some people take great joy in physical labor, especially those whose bodies move naturally, with ease of movement and the enjoyment of innate strength and flexibility. At the end of a day's work, they may feel less worn out than someone who struggled to sit comfortably at a desk all day and then fought traffic to get home. Indeed, upward mobility can often spell the end of natural mobility. How many people do you know who suffer from ill health because of a lack of physical activity? Even people who regularly exercise and work out in the hopes of counteracting a sedentary lifestyle will often pay someone else to mow their lawns.

I sometimes imagine what it would be like to live in a community where citizens engage physically in community life by helping their elderly neighbors clean leaves from their gutters, by growing food in large, thriving community gardens and participating as partners alongside local government workers to maintain the roadsides and public facilities. Where I live, we spray poison on the weeds along the sides of our roads, a quick-fix way of dealing with not having the human resources to do it otherwise. This practice is both unhealthy and unsightly. Dealing with the problem of roadside weeds could be a great form of exercise for many people who could simultaneously practice how to bend and lift in natural, comfortable ways!

Making choices like these are one more part of creating the kind of world we want to live in by choosing to live it that way ourselves.

INTRODUCTION

If you currently experience aches and pains that you accept as a natural consequence of having a body or as an inevitable feature of growing older, you may be surprised at how much more comfortable you can learn to be. If you jog, weight-train, engage in stretching programs such as yoga or participate in sports, you may find that some aspects of these activities require effort and struggle or leave you feeling discomfort afterwards. It is likely that you can learn to eliminate much, if not all, of this struggle and discomfort by changing the way you sit, stand, bend, walk—even sleep.

If this sounds like some sort of simplistic, over-blown claim, I can say I would have agreed with you before I came upon a body education and movement technique called Balance. Until 1997, when I began to study with Jean Couch, the founder of Balance, I was a yoga teacher with a rigorous practice who was continually plagued with recurring tension in my neck and shoulders and a back condition that could be relieved only by daily stretching. Unfortunately, stretching sometimes aggravated a hip that was unstable and "popped" out of alignment in certain positions and activities.

In spite of the fact that for a number of years I had been teaching other people how to relax (proving the adage that you teach what you need to know), I held on to varying amounts of tension in my body and my mind. I was generally unaware at the time that I was doing this. I also didn't realize that I had become addicted to stretching and working out. After all, wasn't I doing what other conscious people were doing—taking care of myself by working at staying fit? Because stretching and sweating away tension felt so good and gave me such relief, I never questioned why the tension returned again so quickly or why I had to repeat my exercise regimen on a daily basis. When I skipped the stretching for any reason, the aches and pains returned in no time at all.

Of all the species on earth, only humans appear to be subject to injury and strain while engaging in normal, everyday activities. In an age of highly sophisticated technological achievement, 80% of the people in America suffer back pain at some point, the total cost of treatment for which tops $100 billion a year. Spinal fusion surgery, a costly ($35,000) radical treatment, jumped 77% in the United States between 1996 and 2001. Even some doctors who perform these surgeries are looking for less invasive solutions since surgical outcomes can be less than desirable, resulting in too many cases of nerve damage, infection or just plain lack of improvement. Epidural steroid injections can, in the best cases, block out pain for months at a time and are fast becoming the new quick-fix approach to back pain. Less invasive than surgery, epidurals still pose risks, including rare though real side effects, and offer only temporary relief at best. Yet, people are lining up to undergo these procedures, so desperate are they to find relief from their pain.

Added to the high incidence of back pain are other kinds of pain from which many people suffer— pain in the neck, jaw, head, shoulders, wrists, hips, knees and feet. Replacing joints has become commonplace, and doctors are challenged to find ways to bring relief to their patients now that some of the most relied-upon medications for treating pain have been removed from the market.

What could be causing all this pain?

Some say it is a lack of exercise; others say it is too much or the wrong kind of exercise. Still others say it is bottled-up emotions or the stress of modern living or poor genes or simple bad luck.

Remarkably, the most common cause of pain in the body—postural misalignment— is something that is thoroughly misunderstood by almost everyone in our part of the world. It turns out that our widely accepted belief about what constitutes good posture is based on faulty information that can lead directly to much of the pain we experience. Not realizing that our bones are designed to hold us up, we rely on muscles to do that job instead, a situation that creates a whole chain of events that ends with P-A-I-N. This mistaken view is so widespread in our society, so thoroughly entrenched in our bodies and our minds, that it pervades almost every system of exercise, almost every belief about fitness and many of the messages we receive from doctors, other health professionals, exercise teachers and sports coaches.

No one, of course, is at fault for this. Such is the way of cultural conditioning, where a collective hypnosis takes hold over the course of many years and puts nearly everyone under a spell based on faulty assumptions. In our current cultural milieu, many of our assumptions about health and fitness are built on what we have been taught. Parents, teachers, role models, TV, movies, advertising, magazine covers—all of these have also been shaped by the same mistaken belief of how our human bodies are designed to work. This belief says that muscular strength—i.e., *tension*—is what

PART I
A Body of Knowledge

The miracle is not to walk on water.

The miracle is to walk on the earth in peace.

Thich Nhat Hanh

Chapter One
The Shape We're In
it might not be what you think

Who is more fit? A small woman with elastic muscles and naturally aligned bones or a larger man with "six-pack abs" and firmly developed pectorals, deltoids and biceps?

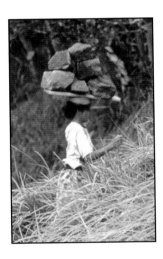 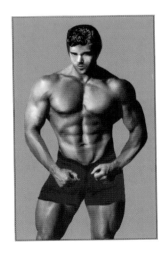

The small woman pictured here is able to carry heavy rocks on her head all day long without strain. Because her bones are aligned and doing most of the work of carrying the rocks, her muscles are able to relax as well as contract, a key component of true fitness.

The man pictured here is clearly strong in ways the woman is not. His power lies within his muscles, not in an overall integrated whole of fully functioning parts. The popular culture of fitness today is partly based on the idea that developed muscles are a requirement of fitness. Unfortunately, muscles that have been developed in this way are storehouses of tension, making it difficult for them to lengthen and relax. This type of strength must be worked at continuously and is dependent on a regular maintenance routine. This man's spine is shortened and compressed, and his breathing is restricted by a diaphragm that doesn't move in a natural, efficient way. The range of motion of his shoulders and hips is greatly restricted. It is ironic that the strength he has worked so hard to acquire has also become a type of weakness.

Two Kinds of Strength

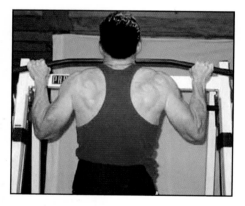

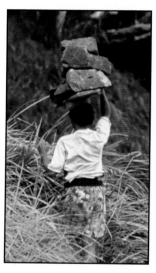

This kind of strength:	This kind of strength:
• has its power in developed muscles.	• has its power in aligned bones.
• must be continuously worked at to be maintained.	• is inherent and is reinforced in ordinary, everyday activities.
• limits the range of motion of the joints.	• is related to open joints.
• shortens and compresses the spine.	• extends the spine.
• restricts elasticity of the diaphragm.	• maintains elasticity of the diaphragm.
• chronically contracts muscle fibers.	• promotes elasticity and relaxation of muscles.

Millions of people live with chronic aches and pain that severely limit their activities, affect their ability to work, cost them thousands of dollars in lost wages and impair their enjoyment of life. Employers, insurance companies and workers' compensation funds pay millions of dollars each year in benefits to injured workers and for lost time on the job.

Whether pain is chronic and low-level or severe and debilitating, it has become an enormous problem in our country. In fact, pain is so commonplace, it has come to be considered normal, something simply to be managed since getting rid of it can be so hard to do. Generally referred to as musculoskeletal pain, it can encompass lower-back pain, arthritis, sciatica, fibromyalgia, plantar fasciitis, temporomandibular joint (TMJ disorder) and chronic tension in neck and shoulder muscles. Much of this pain has no clear, defined cause, making it difficult for doctors to know how to treat it.

When asked what caused their pain, people will often say things such as, "I shouldn't have lifted that box of books." Or "I've been running for 20 years, and my knees finally wore out." Or "I'm not as young as I used to be."

However, if these people knew what their bodies were actually telling them, they might respond with more accurate answers. "Bending to lift a box of books, my pelvis was tucked under, causing my spine to round and forcing my back muscles to strain rather than relying on the strength of aligned bones working with the strength of my legs and arms to do the work." Or, "Running for 20 years with misaligned bones has put persistent stress on my knees, causing the cartilage to wear out." Or possibly, "This aging body is now paying the price for not living according to its natural design."

It can be startling to discover that exercise, in and of itself and in spite of its obvious benefits, is neither the problem nor the solution to this kind of pain in the long run. Eventually, we all pay the price if our bones have not been given the opportunity to do their job of supporting us throughout the years. We will look at ways to exercise safely in Part II.

Musculoskeletal pain is far less of a problem in some parts of the world, even in places where people do a lot of manual labor for years on end. Their secret seems to be that they never lose the biomechanical principles of the human design, something each of us discovered when we first learned how to stand and walk.

The dictionary defines fitness as "possessing a quality of strength and overall health." Nevertheless, for many people today, fitness has become more about how one looks than how one feels. This is a cultural standard that has nothing to do with what is natural to our species' design.

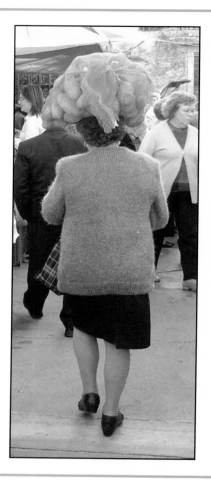

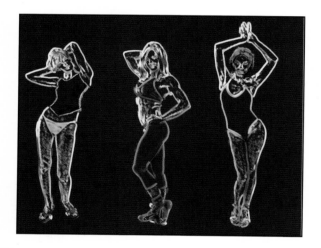

In our popular quest for fitness, many of us unwittingly disregard the importance of skeletal alignment and create conditions that compromise our long-term health. A misaligned skeleton causes chronic muscular tension, thus restricting mobility. It impairs breathing, compresses vertebrae, puts pressure on and distorts the spinal cord (the main neural pathway), affects blood flow and causes chronic muscular tension. It would be hard to argue with the fact that all of these factors have far-reaching consequences for one's health.

Fitness becomes something other than what we thought it was when we apply it to a middle-aged woman who is clearly out of shape by our cultural standards yet easily carries 50 pounds of potatoes on her head. Many people who regularly work out would feel a strain in their backs or necks if they tried to do this. It's probably a safe bet that the woman pictured at left does not exercise at a gym, practice yoga or Pilates, jog, lift weights (except for potatoes on her head) or engage in any other type of formal exercise. Her strength is of a different sort than simply the muscular kind because her bones are aligned in a natural way that has never changed from the time she was a young child. Her strength is neither superficial nor artificial but instead is genuine and truly bone-deep.

There's a kind of fitness that has little to do with something we have to work at, but rather with something we quite naturally happen to be. Being in shape in a natural way has to do with being genuinely stronger, more flexible and healthier than we could ever become by trying to achieve these traits through manufactured means. Being strong, flexible and healthy in this way has to do with being who we essentially are and comes about by inhabiting the body we have as close to its original design as possible.

In America, 80% of people suffer back pain and seek treatment at some point, be it chiropractic, massage, or physical therapy; Rolfing; acupuncture or surgery. The total cost of treating those who suffer back pain tops $100 billion a year. The incidence of back pain drops dramatically in those places where people don't sit at desks all day or consistently use cars and computers or watch televisions. Yet, it is important to note that it is not one's level of activity that determines whether one will experience back pain or not but the position of the bones in relationship to each other. The alignment of the skeleton dictates whether muscles will work in a natural and efficient way or in a way that is prone to pain or injury.

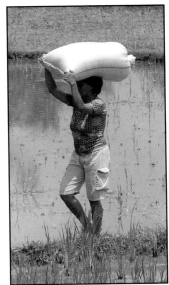

Most people in pain would just like to feel more comfortable. It is hard to imagine that there is a relationship between one person carrying a heavy load on her head and someone else getting rid of pain. Yet, those who carry loads on their heads hold the secret to how to be comfortable and pain-free for those people who have adopted unnatural habits of use over the years. Even lifting weights and otherwise working out cannot prepare one to do this if one's bones are not naturally aligned to begin with. Indeed, muscle development can interfere with a quality of relaxed strength that is essential for living in a comfortable, pain-free body.

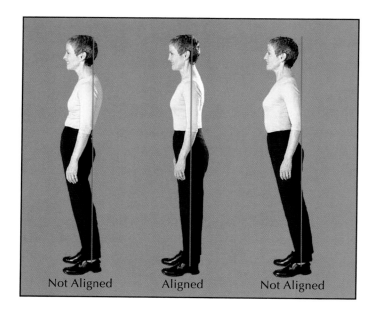

Not Aligned   Aligned   Not Aligned

Each of the red lines added to the figures above begins at the ankle joint and moves upward, similar to the way a building is constructed from the ground up. Only the figure in the middle reveals legs that are vertical along a plumb line and thus able to support the body without tension. This body is divided almost perfectly in half by this line, with all the various body parts—vital organs, blood vessels, muscles, bones—in a naturally prescribed relationship to each other. Most people in technologically developed places would be represented by the figures at one end of the spectrum or the other but rarely in the comfortable middle, where the spine is perfectly aligned and optimally extended.

In an attempt to counteract the effects of our sedentary lifestyle and the slouching that often accompanies it, a culture of exercise and fitness has grown up that emphasizes muscle strength. The question now begging to be answered by serious research is this:

Can someone be truly fit if the spine—the very core of the nervous system—is not aligned along the central axis?

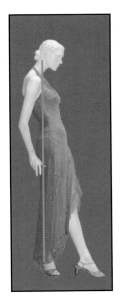 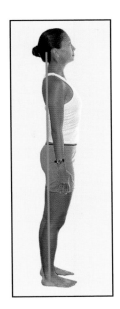

Many factors contribute to the shape we have as well as the shape we're in. Inherited body type and other traits, personal habits, injuries and trauma, cultural conditioning, chronic pain, emotional patterning of muscles, types and levels of activity are all factors that determine our shape. At a very young age, we begin to unconsciously imitate the postures, gestures, styles and tensions of those around us. Before long, we become adolescents and may start to acquire the gestures of our friends and idols. Perhaps without realizing it, we take on a defiant stance or attempt to withdraw, literally, by collapsing into ourselves in the form of slouching or slumping in an attempt to become invisible. Many of these early habits can last a lifetime and can affect our alignment.

Most of us are unaware of the extent to which our image of ourselves and the shape that we take on is defined by others, including the media presentations of certain ideals that are both unnatural and, consequently, unhealthy. This is no one's fault—not even the media's—as we are all lost together in the shadows of our conditioning. It is this conditioning that tells us that while men must present themselves simply as strong, women have primarily two accepted versions of how to inhabit their bodies. One way is the fashion-model stance (above left) with the pelvis tilted back, the hips and legs extended forward, the upper body leaning behind. The other stance (above right) is more assertive, with the head, breasts and buttocks all held high. Both of these positions require certain muscles to be constantly—and unnaturally—contracted, which often leads to pain and other problems.

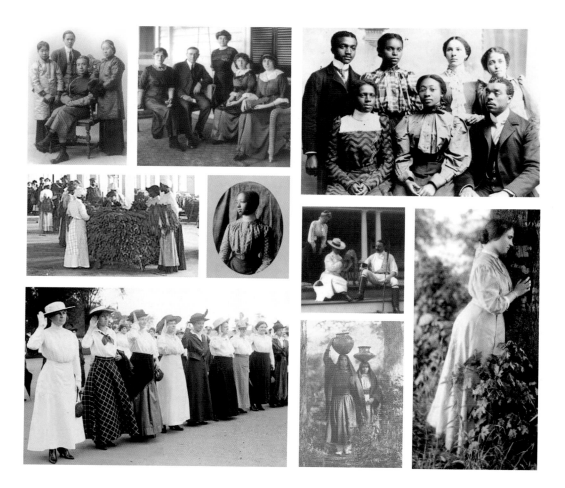

Photographs of early North American life, beginning with the earliest Native Americans and including peoples from other countries, who came to live in the United States, reveal many naturally aligned bodies. Historical photographs show that many people up until the early part of the 20th century lived with their skeletons lined up along the natural plumb line. While the style of dress was more formal back then, the people pictured here are not rigid or stiff but instead are naturally relaxed and noticeably upright.

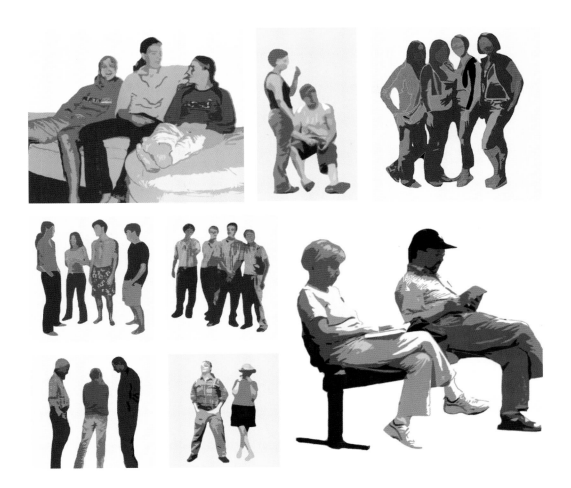

A glimpse inside a photo album today reveals bodies that typically no longer stand or sit in a naturally aligned way. For the most part, even when people are trying to stand up straight, their legs are seldom perpendicular in the way they need to be to provide adequate support for the upper body. Many changes have occurred during the past century, with great advances in many areas. Cultural changes have led to a less formal way of life, including style of dress and ways of inhabiting the body. Unfortunately, along the way people have generally forgotten how to inhabit natural, aligned bodies, which may account for the disproportionately high number of people facing back pain and joint replacement surgeries in the technologically developed parts of the world today.

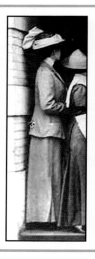 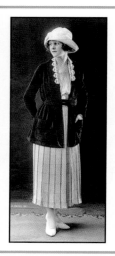 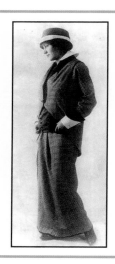 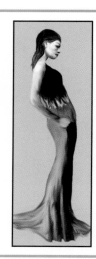

In the United States as well as in some other technologically developed parts of the world, the progression from being naturally strong and upright might look something like this, with the woman on the far left standing in a natural way. Fashion and fads have driven many changes in posture. Now, in the 21st century, so many people are suffering cultural memory loss that we have completely forgotten what the natural carriage of a healthy woman looks like and how inherently capable she is of standing on her own two feet (in this case, vertical legs). A healthy woman doesn't have to work at becoming strong. She simply *is* strong. The more she aligns herself with the natural features of her biomechanical design, the more she brings forward her inherent qualities of strength, flexibility, balance and good health—in other words, true fitness.

While men are not at the mercy of fashion trends in the same ways women are, the broader society has expectations for how men should look. There is no socially accepted slouching option for men the way there is for women. Men's efforts to comply with the cultural standard—strong, confident, successful—often prevent them from being comfortable, relaxed and pain-free.

At various times in the past in certain cultures, women's bodies have been constrained by corsets and girdles that, among other things, served to impair breathing, compress internal organs and hold women's bodies captive. While free of such restrictive clothing today, many women are unaware that by sucking in their bellies and lifting their chests up high in order to comply to a culturally

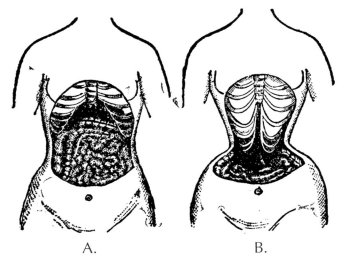

A.   B.

Nature verses Corsets, Illustrated

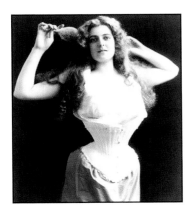
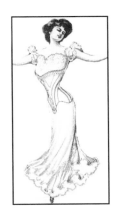

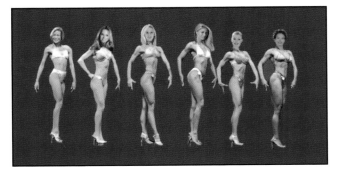

imposed ideal appearance—or alternatively, sink into a fashionable collapse—they mimic, to a lesser extent, some of the same conditions brought about by their great-grandmothers who once wore corsets.

Americans in a multi-ethnic society are all born into human bodies that share the same basic design as those of everyone else. The biggest differences among humans are cultural, geographic, religious and economic but not physical. We speak different languages and have different traditions; we eat different foods and have different religious practices; but, physically, we are all designed to move the same way, using the same muscles to move the same bones. Regardless of our inherited size and shape, we all are meant to sit, stand, bend, walk and even sleep in ways that match the human design. It's the same mechanical system of pulleys and levers that operates inside each individual, regardless of ethnic or racial origin, political or religious affiliation, or basic body

13

type. Culture, however, does affect the physical. Any cultural conditioning, such as the messages we learn about what we *should* look like, has the power to take us away from remembering what is natural to us. Even the design of our furniture and the seats in our cars recondition us away from natural use of our bodies. The reason this all matters so much is that this departure from what is natural often results in pain and poor health.

During my photographic research for this book, I became increasingly aware that people who are the "in" examples of natural alignment live in far greater numbers elsewhere in the world. Many of the "out" examples—those people who no longer are in alignment—are Westerners. As more and more cultures become Westernized, which is occurring today at a rapid rate, we face the serious problem of forgetting en masse how to be naturally human. This unfortunate reality makes the case for natural alignment all the more urgent.

In spite of our many technological advances and remarkable achievements, many of us modern-day Americans, whatever our ancestry and through no fault of our own, have not only lost our ability to inhabit natural bodies but have ended up confused about what good health and fitness really are. If we are to be truly healthy and get ourselves back into shape, we must align ourselves, literally, with the most basic biomechanical features of our design.

The good news is that by examining how some people still use their bodies in a natural way, we can learn to apply universal biomechanical principles to find greater ease and comfort in our own bodies in everything we do.

Chapter Two
Design for Life
every species has its own

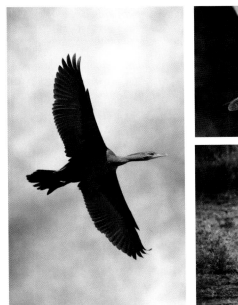
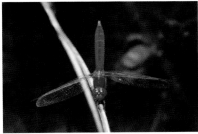
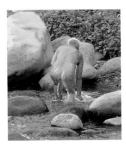
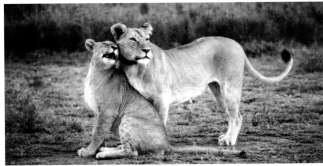

Can you imagine a bird straining its wings from flapping them too hard or a monkey throwing out its shoulder while swinging from branch to branch? How about a giraffe wrenching its neck reaching for a leaf on a tall tree? It seems unlikely these types of injuries ever occur unless an accident happens, such as when a branch breaks while a monkey is swinging on it or a bird is fooled into thinking a glass window is not there. This is lucky because there are no chiropractors or massage therapists, no orthopedic surgeons or personal trainers in the wild animal kingdom.

Every species comes with its very own biomechanical design that defines how it lives. If a bird flaps one wing just a little bit harder than the other one, it will be doomed to fly around in circles. Survival would be difficult.

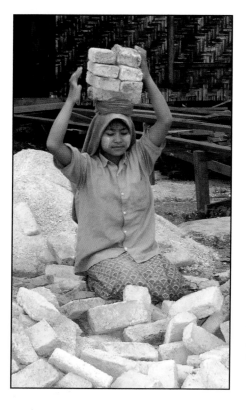

Humans Adapt

Humans adjust to demands put on us by influences in our environment. These could be anything from sitting at a computer all day to following examples set by our parents or the culture in which we grow up. Unfortunately, adapting like this comes with a high price, and we pay for it with a long list of painful consequences.

Only certain humans appear to be prone, in ever-increasing numbers and at younger and younger ages, to throwing out and straining their backs, necks, shoulders, knees, hips, ankles and wrists while engaging in ordinary everyday activities.

This young woman carries bricks and rocks for a living. After loading them on her head, she moves from kneeling to standing with very little effort.

The human body is designed to be remarkably strong and flexible in almost all activities. Many people exclude themselves from believing this to be true for them, thinking they are too weak, too stiff or too old to do anything about it. In reality, from the first moment we begin to apply the same principles used by a small woman carrying rocks on her head, we begin the journey towards being stronger and more flexible—and younger in body.

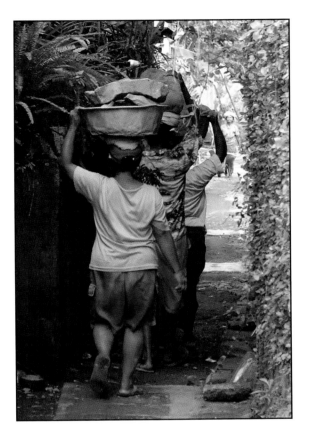 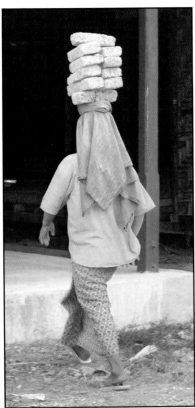

How can it appear so effortless to carry such a heavy load on one's head? The people pictured here are exactly the same species as every one of us, with the same biomechanical design. Most people in technologically developed places would find this a difficult and potentially painful experience, yet these women seem to practically glide through space, in spite of the weight of rocks and bricks bearing down on their heads and spines.

There is no hidden secret to why some people are able to perform strenuous tasks such as these with general comfort and ease. The women pictured here have maintained an ability to inhabit their bodies in keeping with this natural design from the time they were young children.

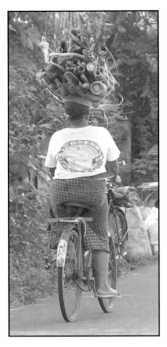 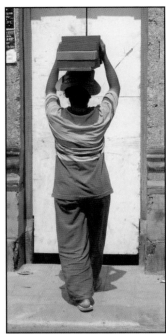 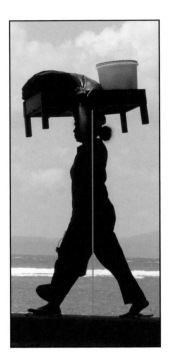

It is a commonly held notion that the human design is faulty, that we have evolved imperfectly (as if this were even possible), and that our spines are not up to the task of supporting us in an upright posture. To think of ourselves as innately flawed suggests that we are apart *from*, rather than a part *of* nature. Such a view ignores the fact that almost anyone can learn once again, with practice, what we all once knew about being aligned and relaxed. As we return to knowing what is natural, the benefits become obvious in how much more consistently comfortable we feel.

Most people who carry things on their heads are able to do so precisely *because* they inhabit their bodies in a wholly natural way. This explains why a middle-aged woman, who appears to be out of shape by our cultural standards, is able to balance a load of wood on her head while easily riding a bicycle. Not only do these people give the appearance that this is effortless—for them, it *is* effortless.

> **A common characteristic of people who live in their bodies in a naturally aligned way is the ease and freedom of their movements, even when they are performing physically challenging tasks.**

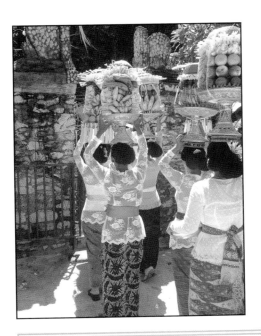

While the spine is not "ageless" in a literal sense (obviously, we all wear out sooner or later), the spine's ability to withstand the forces of gravity and other stresses that accelerate aging are greatly enhanced when we are fortunate enough to be naturally aligned throughout our lives. This is true even when we engage in heavy labor over the course of many years, provided we live by the rules of our design. Indeed, being physically active from a naturally aligned stance reinforces and maintains our basic flexibility and strength and contributes to a level of genuine, easy fitness.

We may have heard it said that people who carry heavy loads on their heads suffer spine and neck damage. This is only true for those who have forgotten how to be aligned with the body's natural design.

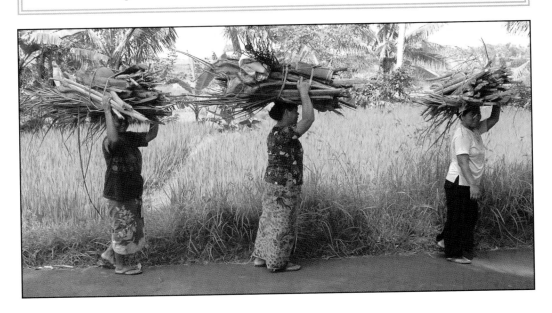

Babies and Young Children as Teachers of Alignment

For those of us who have forgotten how to live in our bodies in a natural, aligned way (read "almost all of us in technologically developed places"), babies become our teachers. This is because healthy children instinctively teach themselves how to turn over, sit up, stand and walk by applying the most basic rules of physics and engineering. If we observe the way babies live in their bodies, we discover what we need to know to return to our natural "home base."

Each one of us is likely to have discovered these laws of our design early in our lives. Through no fault of our own, we gradually became conditioned away from knowing what is natural to us. Many of us have forgotten that our physical being as humans is deeply set in the natural world, governed by the same laws that apply to all life on this planet. Why would humans, who also live on this planet, be any exception to these rules?

When learning to stand and walk, a baby discovers the crucial middle point—the central axis—around which its body organizes itself with exquisite symmetry. This places the bones where they belong and relieves muscles from having to work to hold up the body.

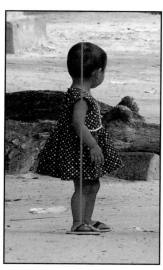 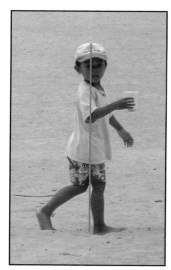

Many of our physical complaints, be they pain or illness, might well be related to a no-blame ignorance of the most basic rules of nature.

It's the Bones, Baby

By the time a baby is ready to walk, she has done the work of training her legs to be well-prepared to support her. For months she has held onto a chair leg or someone's hand and bounced up and down thousands of times. She's learned, through a process of trial and error, to find the positional relationship between leg bones, pelvis, sacrum, rib cage, spine and skull that best supports her quest to be vertical. Why, then, we might ask, is she teetering so tentatively as she works up the courage to drop Daddy's hand and take that first momentous step on her own? Simply put, she's discovering *balance.*

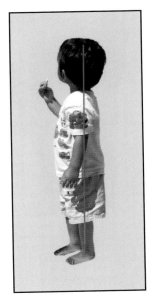

A baby's greatest challenge in learning how to walk is finding how to balance a very large and heavy head on top of the spine, much like balancing a bowling ball on the end of a stick. In this case, however, it's not just a stick but an intricate collection of articulating bones and muscles that must be in correct relationship with one another. Discovering the pivot point where the skull balances delicately on top of the spine allows the neck to be relaxed. While babies may make use of a wider base of support in their legs when first learning to walk, alignment along the vertical axis, for those who are fortunate enough, will remain intact throughout their lifetime.

Relaxation is the key to easy balance, and babies are the gurus of how to live in relaxed bodies. They are able to do this because they have come to understand through experience the exacting interplay between elastic muscles and aligned bones. Babies never stop trying to figure out how things work, including themselves. Seldom is their playing just a random event but rather a natural drive to understand the details of their design.

> **People who never lose what they knew as babies are more apt to live comfortable, pain-free lives regardless of their age, culture, race, body type or level of activity.**

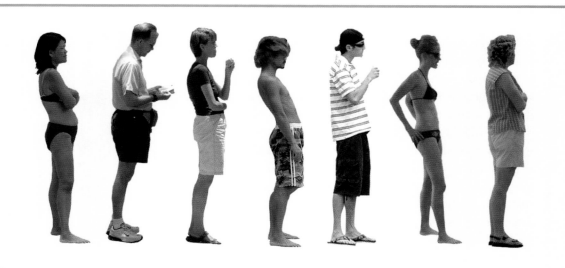

These people are a typical cross section of young to middle-aged people found in America today. It is probably a good thing that none of them is ever likely to want to carry heavy loads on their heads, as their misaligned bones would not be up to the task. Unfortunately, their misaligned bones are not up to the task of holding them up in just about anything that they do, with or without rocks on their heads. It is fairly predictable that most, if not all, of these people experience pain and stiffness on a somewhat regular basis, problems that will only continue to multiply as the years go by. Even if they are able to find temporary relief by stretching muscles, the results must be repeated in an ongoing way until they learn to align their bones. Until their bones end up where they belong, whether they encounter pain and stiffness in their bodies on a daily basis, they will develop problems on an ever-escalating scale in the years ahead.

As very young children first learning how to walk, every one of these people discovered for themselves how to align their bones in keeping with our species' design. In the years that followed, a variety of habits were imposed on them, for many different reasons, that set particular patterns of use into place, much the way default settings are established in a computer program.

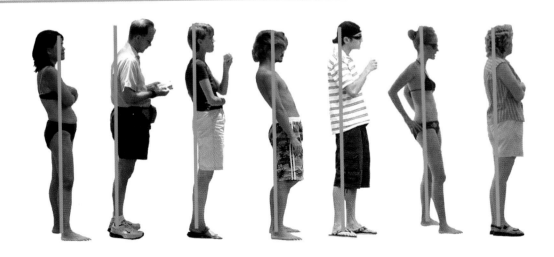

When we observe these bodies once again, this time with a line drawn upward from the ankle, we see that they no longer line up along the central axis in the way they all did when they were young children. Instead, these bodies are all displaced from the central axis. This is true of the majority of people in America and other developed parts of the world today. In each one of these bodies, muscles must compensate for the fact that, rather than pillar-like foundation posts, these legs do not offer much support. This causes an entire series of compensations in the body above, all which spell trouble. The arrangement of their skeletons applies to everything these people do, whether it's to stand in line at the bank, sit in a chair, bend to tie their shoes, reach for a book on a high shelf, jog around a track or lift a basket of laundry. These simple actions performed in an unnatural way over and over again, day in and day out, not only determine how they feel today but how they will age tomorrow.

> Carrying heavy loads on our heads is not the goal. Lining up our bodies along the central axis is the goal that will lead us towards natural strength, flexibility, enhanced stamina and greater ease and comfort in our bodies. We do this by learning from those who carry things on their heads without injury or pain.

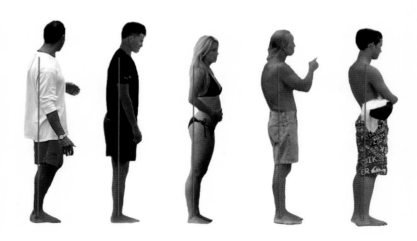

Each one of the people pictured here is an accomplished surfer. In spite of the athleticism they all share, only one of them, the man **second from the left**, stands on leg bones that serve as strong, perpendicular columns. Just as they did when he was a young child, these leg bones support the pelvis in a neutral position that is conducive to a naturally straight and optimally lengthened spine. As a surfer, his ability to balance and move in a fluid way is particularly useful. In the unlikely event that he should ever want to carry a heavy load of rocks (or surfboards) on his head, he would probably be able to do so with relative ease. As an adult with a naturally aligned body, it is improbable that this man will ever lose this basic, albeit unconscious, understanding that all his activities are done in an aligned way and serve to reinforce his natural body condition.

The other four bodies are displaced forward of the line, meaning that muscles are doing the work intended for the bones. As athletes, these people are especially prone to injury from shortened muscles that prevent joints from functioning within a full range of motion.

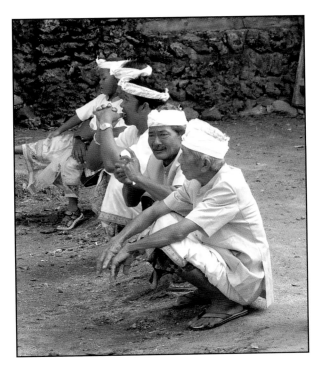

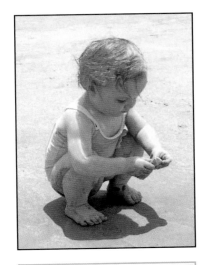

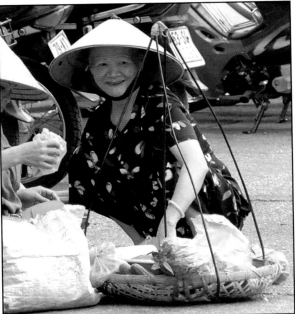

Babies and adults both make use of an identical system of pulleys and levers (muscles and bones). The older people pictured here are an example of how we can remain strong, flexible and comfortable throughout our lives.

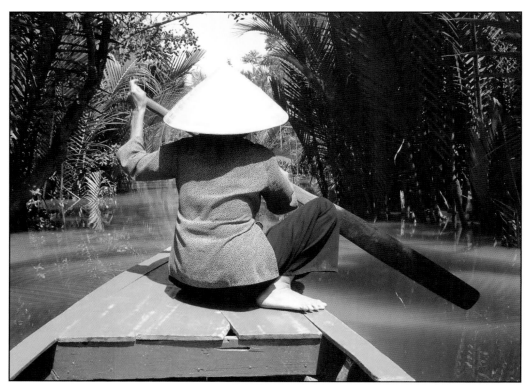

Instead of having to work at building strength and flexibility, we acquire these qualities as natural byproducts of living according to our body's design. Rather than having to engage in a persistent regimen of working out to maintain fitness and muscle tone or pursuing stretching programs to relieve tension stored in muscles, we can simply reinforce our natural strength, flexibility and *length* in everything we do—walking up stairs, playing sports, bending over to feed the cat, vacuuming the house, carrying our groceries, weeding the garden, sitting at the computer or paddling a canoe. It is not a matter of *what* we do but *how* we do it that determines the long-term consequences. Real fitness reflects our naturally aligned and relaxed state.

Putting into practice the principles that will be learned in Part II will allow our muscles to return gradually to their natural length and elasticity. It is not necessary that we all be able to squat in the way that the woman pictured here is doing or to carry heavy loads on our heads. It is enough to learn ways to inhabit the body that let go of tensions that systematically, over time release compressed joints—most especially those of the spine. Doing so will lead us toward a level of natural fitness that will serve us for a lifetime.

Chapter Three
Amazing Grace
carried into old age on a healthy spine

Chances are good that if you live in a technologically developed part of the world, you will not run across many senior citizens who have elongated spines like the ones pictured here.

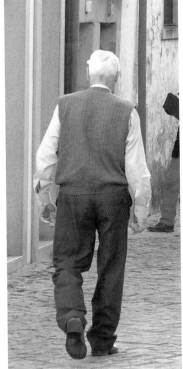

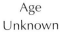
Age
Unknown

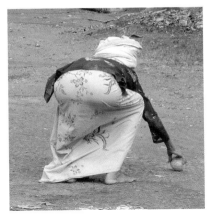

93
Years Old

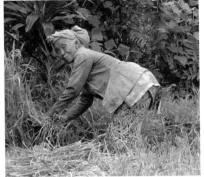

86
Years Old

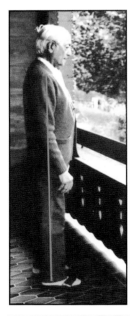

85 years old

Age unknown

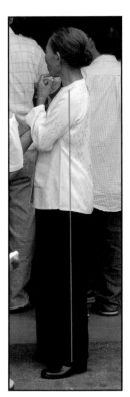

In the same way that young children's bodies line up along the central axis, these people's bodies are divided almost perfectly in half by the axis many decades later.

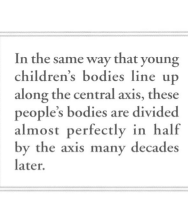

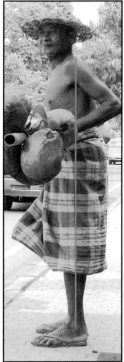

76 years old

92 years old

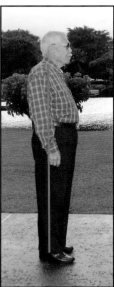

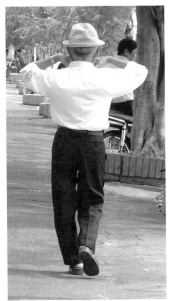

When we enter our later years with an optimally extended, supple spine, the transition is likely to be less abrupt. While we will no doubt be slowing down, we are more likely to have relatively relaxed shoulders, flexible hips, lightness in our step, a natural store of energy and fewer aches and pains.

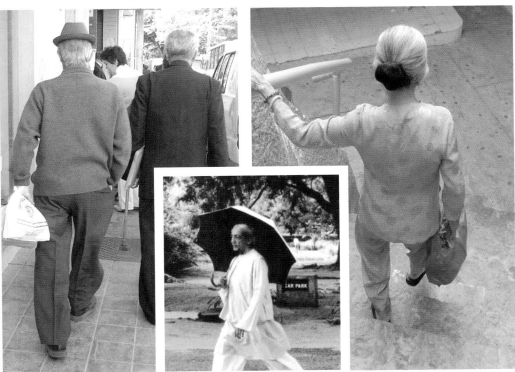

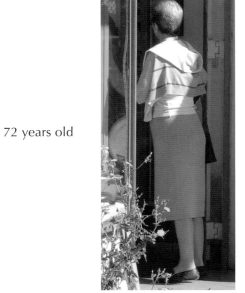

72 years old

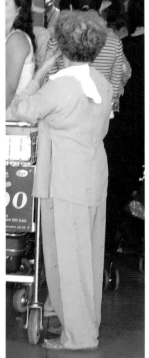

Age unknown

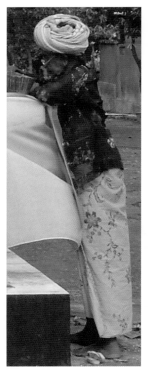

93 years old

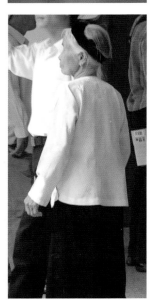

84 years old

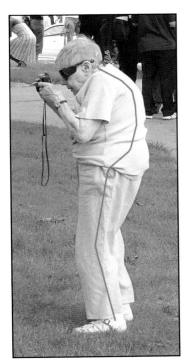
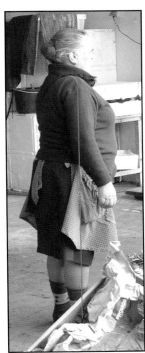

Not long ago, people thought that how one aged was simply the luck of the draw. Some people seemed to have all the luck and managed to move into old age still standing tall and feeling far more comfortable with their bodies. They may have found themselves stiffening up a little bit, but all in all, their bodies didn't cause them a lot of problems. These people glided into old age more gently than those other folks who seemed doomed to follow gravity's commands, sinking into collapsed shapes that left them aching and stiff much of the time.

In recent years studies have clearly determined that inactivity plays an important role in whether people age with greater ease or not. "Use it or lose it" has become the motto of the senior citizen exercise set; the relief many people feel when they become more active bears out what is true about this slogan. In the future, however, as research continues to examine what contributes to healthy aging, it may well come to light that *how* our skeletal structure is aligned in the first place may be even more important than the degree to which we are active. In other words: ***How you use it is how you keep it!***

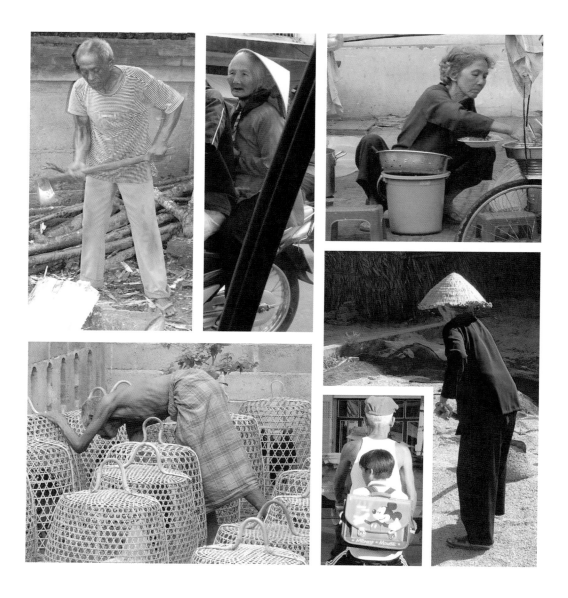

People who maintain natural alignment and supple spines throughout their lives often seem to take pleasure in remaining physically active well into old age. While certain economic realities require that some people work longer, in many instances the concept of retirement is a foreign and unwelcome one.

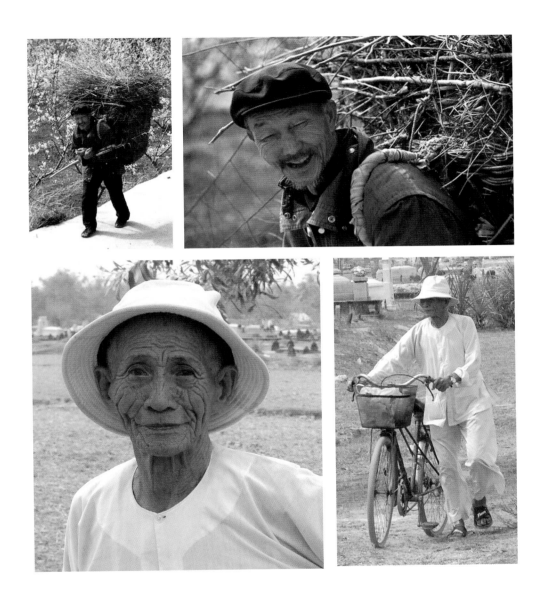

Each of these men has a strong, youthful body for his age. Their genuine and enduring strength and flexibility do not come from developed muscle strength but from living with aligned bones, relaxed muscles and free, open joints.

Chapter Four
Architecture in Flesh and Bone
a moveable spine at the core

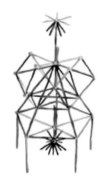

The human body is a living, breathing, walking, talking skyscraper of sorts. Like a skyscraper, it makes use of many of the same architectural principles of compression and tension that work to keep a skyscraper from falling over. This is only one part of the story, however. What makes it possible for a human body, which is not planted firmly in one place but can move about and take on many different positions and withstand the forces of gravity, are structural principles characteristic of *tensegrity*. First described in the 1950s by inventor and engineer Buckminster Fuller, a structure exhibiting tensegrity adheres to an architectural system in which structures stabilize themselves by balancing counteracting forces of tension, as seen in this model made from a popular toy construction set. Whereas a skyscraper is built by employing engineering principles of compression that use the force of gravity meeting the earth through steel structural posts, a tensegrity model emphasizes equally applied tension throughout to offer support.

In architectural terms, *tension* is the result of two parts being pulled in opposite directions from the center, while *compression* is the action where two parts are pressed together from the ends. Think of guy wires used to stabilize a young tree or the Golden Gate Bridge, and this over-simplified explanation will give you the idea. In the tensegrity model of the human design, bones act like spacers between various parts of the body that are joined together by soft tissue—muscles, fascia, tendons, ligaments. This structural system works well for humans as long as there is a balance between the two forces of compression and tension.

Confusion can arise because when we refer to muscular "tension," we usually mean the opposite, in that a muscle shortens (contracts) between its two ends. These two opposite meanings of tension can be addressed by remembering that the essential underlying quality of both kinds of tension is *elasticity,* which is the ability to return to or maintain an original shape and size after being stretched. The tensile forces in engineered structures require elasticity in order to avoid either rigidity or slackness, and muscular tension is almost always an impairment of a muscle's elasticity.

We are far more complicated than any building or bridge, no matter how elaborate its construction might be. We are infused with a life force that animates us and transcends the mechanistic details that, without which, would leave us as nothing more than robots. Rather than perceiving ourselves only as physical objects that think and feel, walk and talk, we may experience ourselves as energy, awareness, spirit-in-action, children of God or simply having a sense of being. We may at times experience the body dissolving away into the emptiness of pure consciousness, beyond all identification, beyond all form. However, it might be that we can experience ourselves at any given time as long as consciousness remains tethered to a physical body—an inseparable one third of the body/mind/spirit triad—and we must play by the rules of physics, all of which in turn are governed by the laws of gravity. We know only too well the stiff neck and backache along with a seemingly endless list of complaints we can experience when we do not play by these rules.

The human design incorporates many basic principles of engineering and architecture that work to help us fulfill our needs for movement as well as withstand the forces of gravity and other stresses. Our musculoskeletal system operates as a basic system of pulleys (muscles) and levers (bones), not unlike a construction crane. Humans have borrowed from their own ingenious design. They have created a variety of mechanical inventions that operate using systems of pulleys and levers, employing principles of tension and compression in addition to modeling ball-and-socket and hinge joints that allow for efficient bending, rotating and pivoting of mechanical parts.

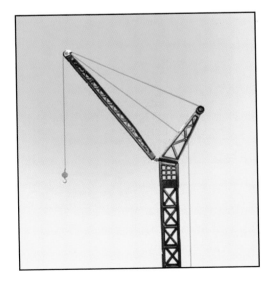

The problem with the tensegrity model is that we tend to fall into the trap of thinking that muscles and other soft tissue do the work of holding us up. This is only true when bones are misaligned and muscles are forced into an exaggerated state of tension to compensate for the lack of proper alignment. In spite of the obvious supporting role that muscles do play, it is important to remember that their primary function is to move bones. A healthy muscle is elastic, able to contract on command and, free of excess tension, able to relax. When bones are placed where they belong, they do most of the work of holding us up and of supporting the weight of whatever it is that we might be carrying.

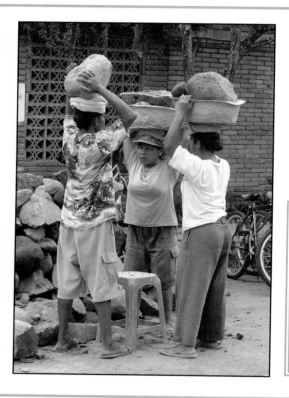

Many of the problems that people experience in their bodies result from the fact that the forces of tension and compression are unbalanced, usually with too much reliance on the tensile aspects of their design.

It makes sense that humans as upright creatures would need a design that makes it possible to withstand the downward pull of gravity and also to counterbalance the tensile forces of muscles and connective tissue. Just as a tall building requires vertical support posts that are strong and perfectly perpendicular to the ground, so do upright *Homo sapiens*. This structure represents a masterpiece of evolutionary design.

Let's Hear It for the Bones

Picture a skeleton, and it conjures up images of Halloween and archaeological finds. Because the skeleton is what remains after all else has disintegrated, we often think of it as a symbol of death or a gruesome collection of lifeless old bones. If this is how you view the skeleton, think again. Right now, there is a living, breathing human skeleton reading these words. The bones that make up your skeleton are dynamically alive, manufacturing blood cells, providing a storehouse for essential nutrients and playing a part in neural and circulatory pathways. Its complex construction includes its ability to withstand extraordinary compressive forces, yet it is malleable enough to undergo a continuous process of being formed and modified, added to and subtracted from throughout the length of one's lifetime.

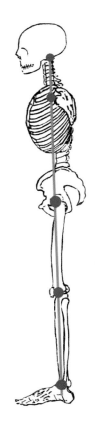

The red line drawn through this skeleton indicates the central axis. This is the same axis that guided each of us as we were first learning to stand and walk. This axis passes directly through the center of the leg bones, the pelvis, the rib cage and the pivot point where the head rests delicately poised on the atlas, the topmost vertebra of the spine. Each weight-bearing joint—ankle, knee, hip, shoulder—rests along this line and is stabilized by muscles that are neither too tight nor too lax. It is this precise alignment of the bones that utilizes their compressive strength, making it possible for some of us to carry heavy loads on our heads. It becomes apparent why it is not brute muscle strength but vertical support from a strong column of bone that bears the weight of the load.

> "Bone resembles steel, with the strength for endurance, substance and stiffness to resist compression and a degree of yielding to sustain shocks. Its resistance to pressure is extraordinary."
> —Mabel Todd, *The Thinking Body,* 1932

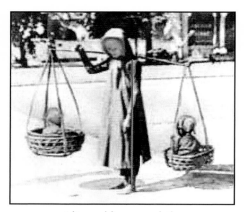

Aligned bones while
carrying two children

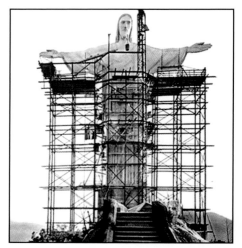

Scaffolding of Christ the Redeemer statue,
Rio de Janeiro, Brazil

We often feel as if we're in a battle with gravity when our bones are not aligned with the vertical reality of our design. In any battle with gravity, gravity always wins. Only by aligning the bones can we withstand gravity's downward pull over the course of many years.

Almost everyone would agree that good posture plays an important role in good health. Yet, remarkably few of us know what good posture really is. What we believe to be true about posture is based on what we have all been taught: that we need to stand up straight, with our shoulders back and down, chest up, chin up, belly in, tailbone tucked under. Every one of these actions engages the tensile forces in a way that is not only unnatural to our evolutionary design, but that is counter to the most basic principles upon which we must rely. These actions draw the bones away from the central axis and actually prevent natural, relaxed alignment at a comfortable home base.

Scaffolding as Framework

The central axis divides the aligned body evenly in every direction. Lines drawn through the weight-bearing joints at their points of articulation demonstrate the verticality of our uprightness as well as reveal the scaffold-like framework that applies to our design. Even more reliable and lasting than muscle strength is the strength we have that is "bone deep." We need only imagine the instability that arises in scaffolding if the foundation posts are askew to understand why misaligned bones can eventually lead to joint-replacement surgery.

The human skeleton is an architectural wonder of symmetry and functionality. The fact that its underpinnings are guided by rules of physics and engineering is, in part, what makes it possible for this seemingly rigid structure to move with such freedom and fluidity. Without the resulting support of applying these biomechanical principles, our muscles do most of the work of holding us up. This causes us to expend tremendous energy and is a frequent cause of pain and discomfort.

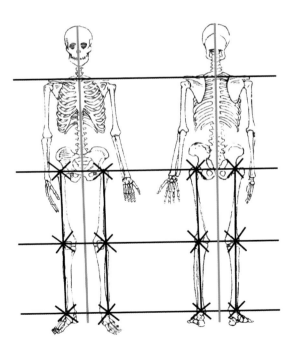

Our cultural tendency to veer off from the central axis may play a big part in helping to explain some of the health issues that are now particularly epidemic in developed parts of the world.

Being aligned is not about being thin. The woman in the middle has a sturdier body type than the others shown here, but she enjoys the benefits of being aligned and relaxed. This raises yet more questions about what real fitness might be. While the benefits of a healthy diet and physical activity are crucial to good health, we tend to ignore the vital role played by natural alignment.

Weight-bearing joints (yellow dots) line up along the central axis.

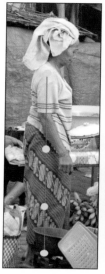 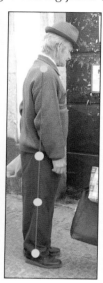 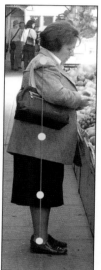 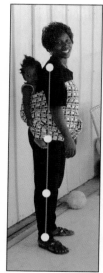 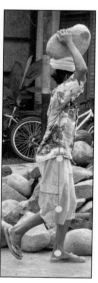

Characteristics that naturally aligned people share when standing

- Leg bones form vertical columns of support.
- Central axis evenly divides the entire body almost exactly in half.
- Weight-bearing joints—ankle, knee, hip, shoulder—line up along the central axis.
- Pelvis and rib cage are in a natural, neutral position.
- Spine is optimally elongated.
- Muscles throughout the body are evenly balanced and elastic.
- Internal organs are positioned naturally and not compressed.
- There is an inclination toward freedom from pain and tension.

These people must lean the upper body backward in order not to fall forward, tightening a whole host of muscles in the process. It is common for people who stand this way to cross their arms or place them on their hips to relieve the subtle pull of the arms hanging out of the shoulders.

The clothes these people wear reveal a lot more wrinkling and creasing of fabric than the clothes worn by the people on the previous page. One can imagine how this relates to the "wrinkling" of organs, veins, arteries and other parts inside the body and how this might affect one's health.

Weight-bearing joints (yellow dots) are unstable and under constant stress

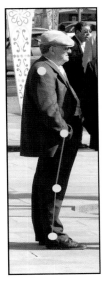 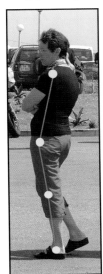 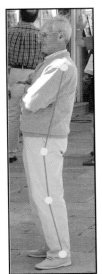 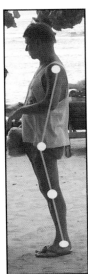 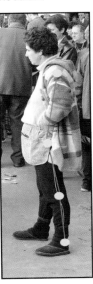

Characteristics that unnaturally aligned people share when standing

- Leg bones are not perpendicular and don't offer solid support to the body.
- No central axis is present along which these bodies line up.
- Weight-bearing joints are not supported one above the other and are compressed and under stress.
- Pelvis and rib cage are misplaced.
- Spine is contracted and shortened.
- Muscles throughout the body are forced to be chronically contracted.
- Internal organs are ill-positioned, crowded and compressed.
- There is an inclination toward experiencing frequent pain and tension.

The Trunk of the Tree and So Much More

The spine is essential to our being upright. Made up of 24 vertebrae and the sacrum on which they sit, the spine is an ingenious construction defined by both stability and mobility. While it is far more complex than a stack of blocks, it does have certain features in common with those blocks. Each vertebra is precisely shaped to land on the one below it, separated by a gel-filled cartilaginous disc that cushions bone from rubbing against bone, enhances movement and provides hydraulic shock-absorbing qualities. The vertebral body gives the spinal column the power to resist compressive forces while a complex arrangement of multifaceted joints gives the spine its ability to be fluid and mobile, not rigid. This gives us the flexible support we need to move with comfort and ease.

Besides giving support to the torso, the spine also supports the skull and provides for its multidirectional movements. The spine's processes serve as anchor points from which the rib cage hangs in a precise arrangement that allows for optimal breathing. The spinal cord, which is the primary neural pathway that sends and receives messages from the brain, is encased and protected within the spinal canal. Optimal functioning depends on the spine maintaining its natural alignment. The old adage "You're only as old as your spine" speaks to the fact that how we age in addition to our overall health and well-being is directly related to the condition of the spine.

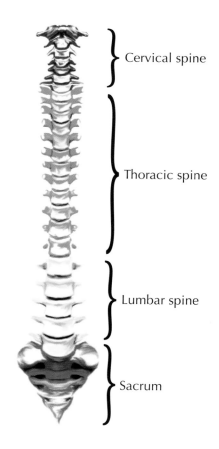

Cervical spine

Thoracic spine

Lumbar spine

Sacrum

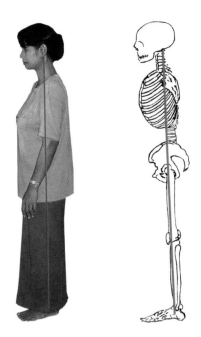

Someone whose skeleton lines up along the central axis will exhibit the following qualities:

- maximum length through the spine
- a neutral position of the pelvis atop vertical leg bones
- a rib cage that hangs naturally from its points of attachment to the spine
- a long extended neck
- a skull that balances on top of it all

Standing for long periods of time this way is not difficult because there are few points of stress to cause discomfort or restlessness.

A common characteristic of people who are aligned like this is the way in which their clothes drape, with hemlines that are more or less level and with an absence of bunching and wrinkling of fabric.

> **People who are naturally aligned, like the women pictured here, do not have the "hard-body" look that is so popular today. Their muscles are elastic and pliable, and their grounded strength comes from the interplay of aligned bones, flexible muscles and open joints.**

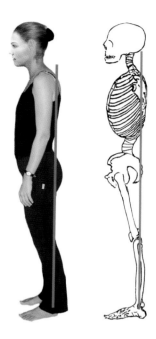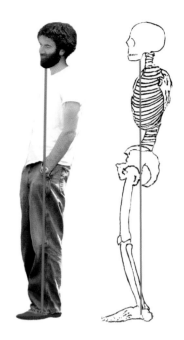

The spine can be distorted away from the center in different ways. The lumbar spine (lower back) of the woman on the left is arched (lordosis), and her skeleton is displaced forward of the central axis, causing a shortening of the spine. The young man's spine is also collapsed in the front; yet, the pronounced backward tilt of his pelvis flattens out the lower back. In the end, the effect is the same for both of these people—a shortened, compressed spine. The inevitable tension and possible pain these people are bound to experience can show up in many places, including the back, neck, shoulders and joints of the extremities.

Relaxing is not the same as slouching or collapsing. True relaxation can only happen when the bones provide aligned support. Only then can the muscles really relax.

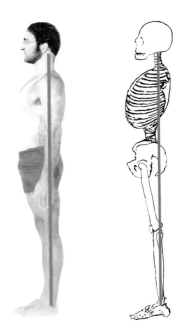

This stance represents the most common attempt to counteract the effects of slouching and collapsing of the chest. Lifting the chest and drawing in the belly, while developing muscle tone to support this position, is what many people believe is an essential ingredient of fitness. Unfortunately, fitness cannot be achieved through chronic misalignment of bones and the tremendous muscular tension required to hold oneself together in this way.

A clear distinction can be drawn between what is "normal" and what is "natural." In order to feel your best—relaxed and pain-free—your spine must be optimally aligned along the central axis, not displaced forward from it and arched and shortened, as seen here.

> **Standing up straight in the way we have been taught actually causes the spine to be arched and compressed**. *This is one of the primary causes of chronic back pain and injury.*

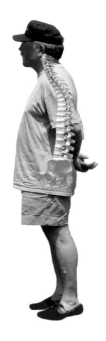 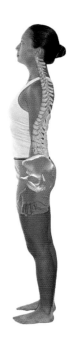 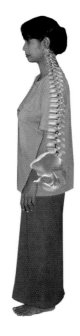

This man's pelvis and sacral platform tilt backward while his upper spine arches forward. This is typical of how many of us stand today and is a prescription for back pain. This shortening of the spine only becomes all the more pronounced with age. It is likely this man is accustomed to experiencing various aches and pains.

When leg bones are not aligned like those pictured here, we often try to offset a tendency towards collapse by literally "lifting" ourselves upward. Tremendous muscular effort is required to do this and causes severe arching in the lower back. We often think the spine has three pronounced curves like the ones seen here, but the spine's curves are actually more gradual than this.

This woman requires little muscular effort to stand upright because her aligned bones are providing most of the support she needs. Her muscles are playing a relatively relaxed supporting role. As described in previous examples, her vital organs, blood vessels and neural pathways are all optimally arranged for healthy and efficient functioning.

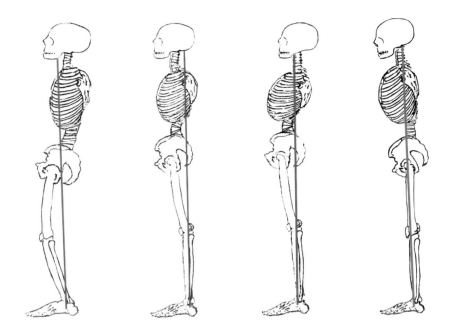

Without adequate support from below, the head bears down heavily on the skeleton on the left, compounding the collapse of the spine. While the skeleton in the middle appears to be more upright, the rib cage is pushed out in front, drawing the spine into a curved bow. This is the chest-up-shoulders-back-abdominals-firm-tailbone-tucked-under approach to standing. It may be normal in our culture, but it is not natural. People who learn how to stand with their bones aligned, as demonstrated by the skeleton on the far right, often report almost instantaneous improvement in addressing tensions or pain they may have struggled with for a long time.

> While a skeleton would never be able to stand on its own without the support of various muscles and soft tissue, it is apparent which one of the skeletons pictured here would have the best chance of standing alone.

We have already seen how easily a relatively small person can carry a heavy load on her head when the vertebrae of the spine are in precise natural alignment. This also relates to the same force/counterforce that allows a bird to fly. As a bird flaps its wings, pushing down on the air, the resistance of the air pushes back up against the bird's wings. If you want to jump high, you have to first drop low. Someone whose spine is naturally aligned will be able to feel a counterforce rising upward through the spine when carrying a heavy load.

Force and counterforce occur naturally in the body when conditions are right. Remarkably, the woman in the photo above is not struggling under the weight of the rocks. If she were trying to resist the downward push with muscular effort, she would be interfering with the balance of forces inherently available to her—internal and external forces would not be equalized, and she

> *For every action there is an opposite and equal reaction.* **Newton's Third Law of Motion (Law of Reaction) means it is possible for small women to carry heavy loads on their heads with ease.**

Heavy load of rocks bearing down through vertebrae

Body of vertebra

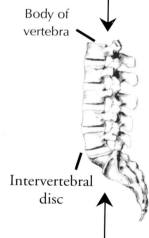

Intervertebral disc

Ground reaction force (GRF) rising upward, generated as opposite and equal reaction

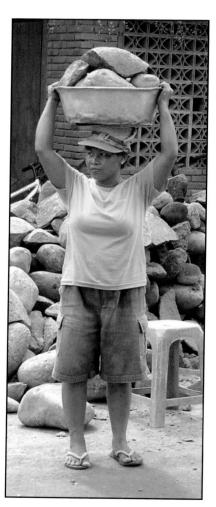

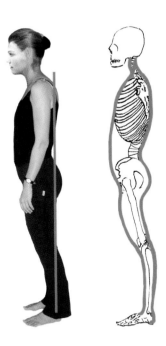 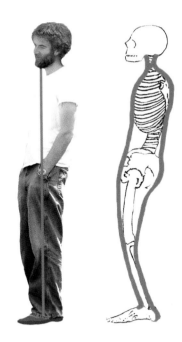

These simplified renderings from a side view reveal how muscle fibers become overly shortened or lengthened when the bones are positioned away from the central axis.

The position of this young woman's bones causes the muscles in her lower back, neck and back of the thighs to tighten, the front of the thighs to overdevelop and the muscles along the front of the torso to overextend. By learning to align her bones along the axis, she can gradually guide these muscles back to their natural length and elasticity.

Elastic muscles are not the same as flaccid, weak muscles. These leg muscles have little opportunity to do their job in standing or walking. Because of the pronounced backward tilt of the pelvis, there is no support for the spine, rib cage or head, which gives the sense of all the muscles sinking downward into a state of collapsed tension.

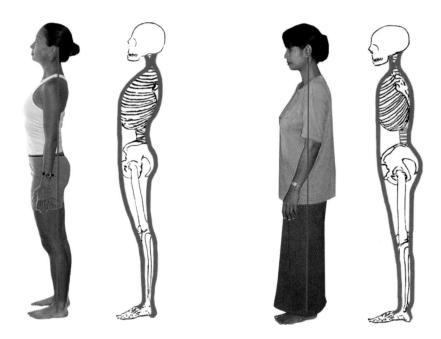

The body on the left may look familiar as representing the ideal upright, athletic and strong woman who works out, plays sports or practices yoga. This particular look is readily seen in magazines and on exercise and some yoga videos.

In this stance, her chest is lifted and her chin and head are drawn back, causing a tremendous tightening of muscles in the neck and all along the spine. This is a rigid position that creates a lot of tension in the body, frequently leading to an urge to stretch on a regular basis.

When the bones are aligned along the central axis, seen in the stance on the right, there is an obvious symmetry to the arrangement of the muscles, which are optimally toned, buoyantly elastic and evenly long. There is very little tension in these muscles and, therefore, no pain.

A Place for Everything and Everything in Its Place

We may not have to keep everything in its place in all situations. But when it comes to the internal workings of the torso, this graphic view makes it clear that the various organs are designed to fit into place in an organized way, much like pieces of a 3-D puzzle.

Our bodies form an intricate relationship between many systems—respiratory, circulatory, endocrine and digestive, to name just a few. It's easy to forget that so much is going on inside of us without us ever having to think about it, whether we are awake or asleep.

The fact that these systems take care of themselves doesn't mean our alignment can't impact their normal, healthy functioning. How well is the liver able to do its job of detoxifying our blood when the rib cage is positioned in such a way as to put a permanent squeeze on it? How efficiently does waste move through the labyrinthine tunnels of the colon if hyper-firm abdominal muscles place constant pressure on them?

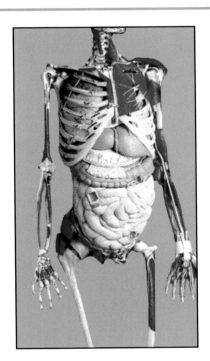

It makes sense that there would be an optimal alignment of the skeleton to support the internal organs in an efficient relationship to each other.

Command Central

> The nervous system is connected to every organ tissue and cell in the entire body. It controls and coordinates all the body's functions, whether they are digestive, respiratory or circulatory and whether they deal with the movement of muscles or how we relate to the world through our senses.

Besides providing structural support, the spine protects the spinal cord within the spinal canal. The spinal cord gathers stimuli from the surrounding environment and relays them to the brain. Instructions are sent from the brain to every part of the body by way of electrical impulses that travel along the spinal cord and subdivide into countless nerve fibers that extend to every corner of the body. When each vertebra is positioned as intended, the impulses can be relayed unimpeded. It seems reasonable that any interference with the normal flow of nerve impulses, including constant distortion of the spinal cord, might affect any part of our bodies, resulting in pain, weakness and difficulties affecting our organs and systems.

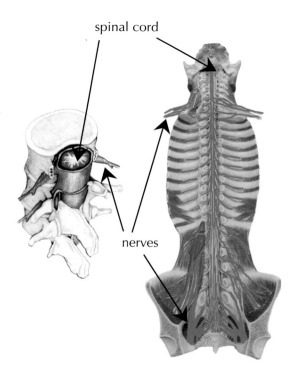

spinal cord

nerves

> The spinal cord is flexible and can be bent along with the spine. "Home base" for the nervous system, just like other systems of the body, lies within a symmetrical center where all the parts are positioned in an integrated relationship to each other for efficient functioning.

Fight or Flight or Just Relax

Independent of the central nervous system is the autonomic nervous system, which is divided into the sympathetic and parasympathetic aspects. The sympathetic nervous system prepares our bodies to deal with emergencies, while the parasympathetic nervous system is the body's vehicle for relaxation, recuperation and renewal. In a healthy and balanced body, both systems work together to maintain homeostasis, a state of equilibrium of the organism.

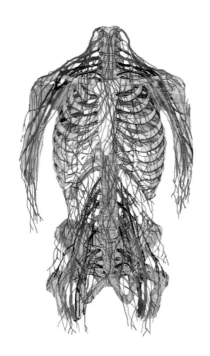

When we are faced with some sort of threat, either real or imagined, the rate at which our hearts beat increases, blood pressure rises, pupils dilate, digestion is stopped and blood is diverted from the skin and viscera to the muscles in preparation for action. If the threat is real, these details help us to respond as needed. Once we have dealt with the emergency, the sympathetic system settles down and the relaxation response kicks in once again. This is a survival mechanism that has been a part of the human race from those earliest of days when our ancestors might have had to escape from an approaching saber-toothed tiger.

In modern life, any number of situations—financial difficulties, traffic jams, job stress, relationship problems—can play a part in engaging the sympathetic nervous system. We get into trouble when it stays "turned on" in a low-level, chronic sort of way. When this is the case, we miss out entirely on the rejuvenating features of the parasympathetic nervous system that are so essential to our health.

> Symmetry of alignment is important for unimpeded transmission of messages and electrical impulses through neural pathways throughout the body.

The parasympathetic nervous system is our natural resting state, marked by a slowed heart rate, lowered blood pressure, increased blood flow to the skin and other organs as well as enhanced digestion and absorption of nutrients. This is a revitalizing state where creativity occurs and where we feel safe, comfortable and relaxed. Engagement of the parasympathetic system facilitates healing and contributes to wellness of our body's organisms. Under ordinary conditions, unless we are faced with a perceived threat, there is no need for the sympathetic system to be dominant.

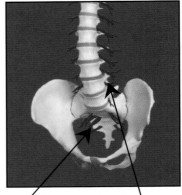

sacral   lumbar nerves

Little research has examined structural alignment of the spine and spinal cord and its affect on the autonomic nervous system (ANS). Since the spinal cord serves as the conduit for neural pathways and initiates engagement of the sympathetic and parasympathetic nervous systems, it makes sense that distortion of the spine through either hyperextension or collapse would affect the free transmission of signals through the spinal cord and ANS nerves. It is reasonable to suspect that chronic skeletal misalignment of one sort or another, over the long term, would prevent the natural state of rest brought about by the parasympathetic nervous system to function in an optimal way. This is a complex scenario that is begging to be examined through research. The possible consequences of this are legion, especially when one considers the relationship of the relaxation response with the health of all the other systems of the body.

> **The fact that there has been no investigation into the relationship between natural alignment and the function of the autonomic nervous system represents a glaring oversight in the field of medical research. Such oversight is understandable, however, given that until now, natural postural alignment has been so thoroughly misunderstood.**

Putting the Parts into a Whole

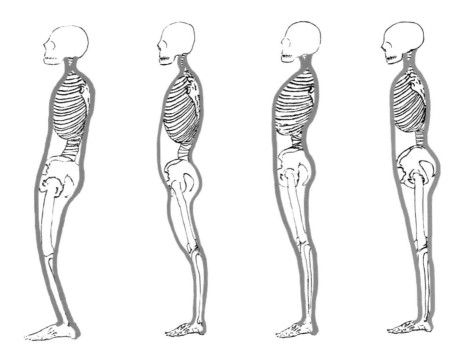

When we revisit these four figures, we can now see more clearly how only one of them (**second from left**) is supported by a strong, stable skeleton with bones in correct relationships with each other. The second figure from the left has an optimally extended spine and joints that are stable and not compressed or under stress. This person also enjoys the benefits of relaxed, supple muscles without stored-up tension and vital organs that are not squeezed together or distorted in cramped quarters. Of the four, this is the only person likely to enjoy the benefits of the relaxation response serving as the home base for the nervous system, rather than the fight or flight response activated at all times.

If the relationship of alignment to the nervous system is not immediately obvious, one need only lift the chest upward while sucking in the belly to experience how this increased muscular tension relates to breathing. Without free, easy breathing, the relaxation response eludes us. The chapter that follows explores this concept in greater detail.

Chapter Five
Three Wheels of Alignment
how do they turn, turn, turn?

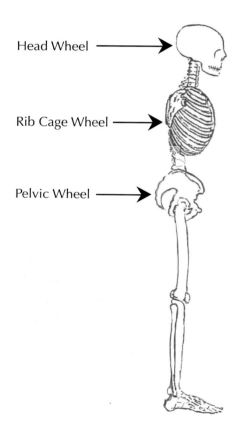

Head Wheel

Rib Cage Wheel

Pelvic Wheel

The concept of the Three Wheels of Alignment gives a clear, visual map that can be translated into the concrete structure that shows how the major bony landmarks of the body relate to each other.

The skull, rib cage and pelvis all share a basic roundness to their shape. Another feature they have in common is that they are all joined together by the spine, beginning at the sacral platform at the pelvis, attaching along the rib cage at the back and traveling up to the pivot point where the skull delicately sits atop the uppermost vertebra. Reducing the 206 bones of the adult skeleton down to its most essential parts, the structure could be described as being made up of three wheels, a spine, two arms and two legs.

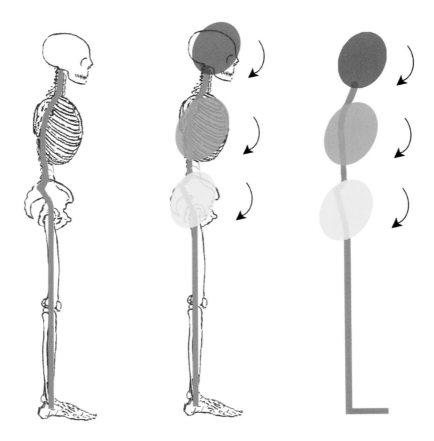

When rounded shapes are superimposed on a naturally aligned skeleton, we arrive at a model that looks like the figure at the right. By designating these shapes as ovals, we are better able to decipher the directions in which they might conceivably move in relationship to each other. In an aligned stance, as the one shown here, we see that all three are turned slightly forward.

This model of forward turning "wheels" of alignment is especially useful for learning how to direct change in the body. Visualizing the wheels and how they turn will help guide the somatic responses that take you through the necessary steps for returning the bones to the central axis.

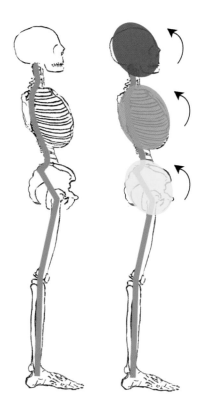

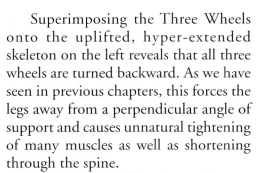

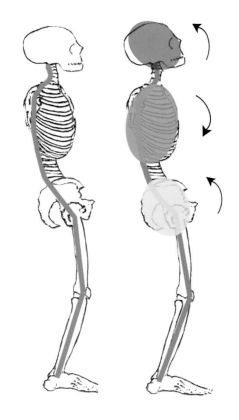

Superimposing the Three Wheels onto the uplifted, hyper-extended skeleton on the left reveals that all three wheels are turned backward. As we have seen in previous chapters, this forces the legs away from a perpendicular angle of support and causes unnatural tightening of many muscles as well as shortening through the spine.

Those who stand like this in whatever degree of backward turning wheels can learn to realign their bones along the central axis by consciously turning the wheels in the other direction.

The collapsed stance shown above involves the Three Wheels moving in different directions from each other, with the head and pelvic wheels rolling backward while the rib cage wheel rolls forward. The spine is compressed and pushed out from the center line by the weight of the turning wheels bearing down on it.

The forward tilt of the rib cage on top of a backward tilted pelvis often causes the legs to buckle from the stress of all the misplaced weight above them.

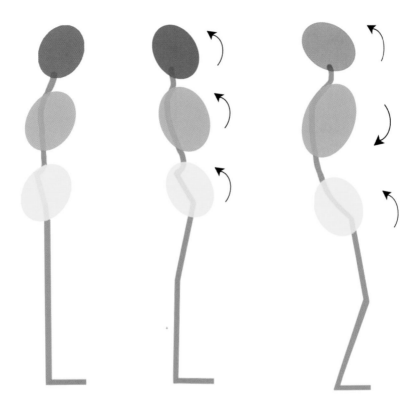

Lined up in a row, these figures demonstrate only three ways of standing. There are numerous other combinations and degrees of wheel directions and leg angles. The more closely the turning wheels bring the skeleton in line with the central axis, the more the body's innate features of being aligned, relaxed, strong, flexible and balanced will fall into place.

No matter how your bones are presently arranged, the basic formula for reclaiming what is natural is the same for almost everyone. Even though muscles are in charge of moving bones, it is not necessary to give them conscious directions. Learning to place the Three Wheels in their most natural relationship with each other is where you start.

Turning the Pelvic Wheel

Muscles respond to the brain's commands without there having to be conscious direction. Unfortunately, when the pelvis is held at an unnatural angle for many years, the muscles have been reconditioned to work in an unnatural way, limiting one's repertoire of movements. For this reason, it can be particularly helpful to initiate any change by focusing on the bones. Consciously guiding the bones to a more natural position in relation to other bones gives muscles an opportunity to gradually change their habits and develop new options that might be more efficient as well as more comfortable.

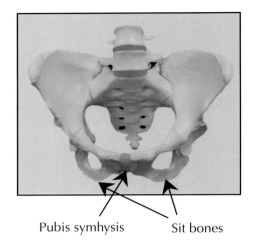

Pubis symhysis   Sit bones

The image of the pelvis as a bowl is one that it often used to describe the possible movements of the pelvis. Pelvis means "basin" in Latin, and while there are obvious similarities, this view of the pelvis can be misleading. A more helpful view is to picture a natural and neutral pelvis as a bowl that is tipped onto its side. The bottom rim now serves to illustrate the way the sit bones perch on a surface when sitting and are

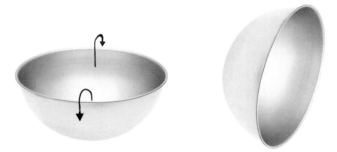

aimed directly downward when standing. This sideways-tipped bowl also captures the oval shape of the pelvic wheel, further demonstrating the direction in which this wheel is turning when it is naturally aligned. In this position, the pubis symphysis is dropping down in front, and the sit bones are wide apart. Old habits sometimes cause arching in the lower back that can be addressed by dropping the chest (i.e., turning the rib cage wheel forward).

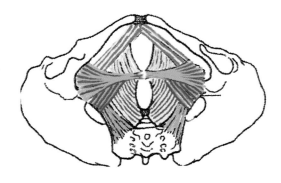

The pelvic floor, because it is so closely tied to tension everywhere else in the body, deserves special attention. It can be difficult to believe that the floor of the pelvis should be relaxed most of the time. Many exercise programs—not to mention cultural messages—tell us that we should tuck our tailbone under and suck in the belly. Suck and tuck. Tucking the tail under is what a dog does when it is cowering, afraid. Indeed, when we tuck our tail under like a dog we feel the floor of the pelvis narrow and tighten, our hips clench and breathing becomes restricted. "Wag your tail" and everything changes—the floor of the pelvis opens up, the position of the pelvis shifts and breathing deepens. (This only works if the rib cage wheel is rolling forward too. More about this to follow).

Think of the floor of the pelvis as a collection of hammocks strung in a crisscross pattern that spans from various attachments at the pelvis. Then, you can also imagine what happens when you squeeze and tighten the configuration of those fibers, pulling and misaligning their natural shape. This is not unlike setting a table with a beautiful tablecloth and fine china and crystal, then giving a tug to one corner of the tablecloth, causing all the table settings to go askew.

Longstanding tension in pelvic floor muscles appears to play a role in some cases of pelvic floor myalgia, prostatitis, interstitial cystitis and incontinence. Allowing these muscles to serve as elastic slings, with their fibers having natural tonus without tightness, helps insure that the pelvic floor stays relaxed. Any pelvic floor exercises a woman does (typically called Kegels) must be done with the pelvis in a neutral position at all times. Further, the muscle movements must be isolated in the floor of the pelvis only, so that there is no tightening of abdominal muscles, drawing upward of the pubis or muscle action in the thighs or buttocks. Placing a hand on the belly and paying close attention to keeping the pubis from moving when tightening pelvic floor muscles will help isolate the movement of these muscles. When done, it is important that the floor of the pelvis returns to being fully relaxed.

Turning the Rib Cage Wheel

Relaxing the belly/abdominal muscles is essential for the rib cage wheel to move independently of the pelvis. Changing the position of the rib cage often causes the pelvis to move as well. This is the result of patterns embedded in abdominal and pelvic muscles that are habituated to unnatural responses. This is not a matter of whether or not one can move the rib cage separately from the pelvis but more a matter of remembering how. To do this, one must release the contraction of more superficial abdominal muscles that act to "glue" the rib cage and pelvis together. Releasing tension in the belly frees up these patterns and allows the bones to move easily in relationship to each other.

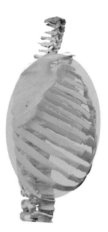
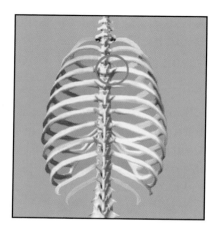

Optimal length of the spine depends on the rib cage being suspended in its natural position from the transverse processes along the side of the spine (see below). Sucking in the belly and/or lifting up the chest, interrupts this free hanging of the rib cage, causing many other muscles to tighten and the spine to shorten. Stabilizing the position of the pelvis and then slowly tightening and releasing the belly can reveal the ways in which abdominal tension interferes with the natural resting place of the rib cage.

With a stable, unmoving pelvis as a foundation, you are also able to investigate how the spine lengthens and shortens along the back when the rib cage wheel is rolled first one way and then the other. We'll look into this more closely in Part II.

Turning the Head Wheel

Most people, when asked where the head and the spine meet, will point to the base of the skull, at the occiput. Yet, when asked to balance a ball on a stick, they place the stick at the center of the ball, not at the edge. Exactly the same principle applies with the head balanced on the spine.

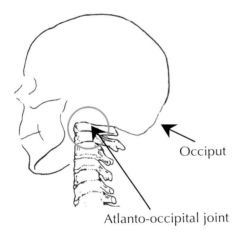

Occiput

Atlanto-occipital joint

If you draw an imaginary line from the tip of your nose out through the back of your head and another line between your ears, the point behind your nose where these two lines intersect is the place where the skull sits on top of the spine. The two uppermost cervical vertebrae, the atlas and the axis, are ingeniously combined as two well-lubricated joints to allow tension-free, relaxed and easy movements of the head and neck.

The jaw (mandible) is not part of the skull but rather an appendage of bone and lower teeth that is attached at a hinge in front of the ears.

The adult head weighs between 10 and 15 pounds. Considering that this is equivalent to a bowling ball, it becomes apparent that with or without a pile of rocks, we are already carrying a heavy load on top of our spines. If you tried to carry a bowling ball with your arms, it wouldn't take long for the arm muscles to tire. Imagine how hard your neck muscles must work to support your head when it is not positioned in its natural way on top of the spine. Many people find great relief from neck and shoulder strain simply by experiencing how their heads are intended to rest on top of the spine.

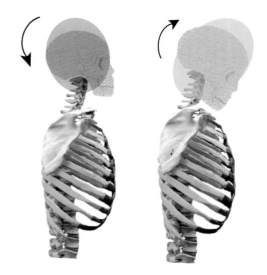

The head can be a heavy burden we struggle to carry around all day. When the chin leads out in front, (figure at left) it sends all the weight into the back of the skull, jamming the head down onto the atlanto-occipital joint. This forces neck muscles to work in ways they are not intended and contributes to headaches, neck and shoulder strain in addition to compression of the spine that affects how one ages.

Looking at the figure on the right, see how turning the head wheel forward allows the spine to lengthen upward. The weight shifts forward into the frontal portion of the cranium as the chin drops toward the chest. Many people find this a difficult concept to accept because we are so thoroughly conditioned to believe the head belongs in the backward-turning position. "Chin up," we're told from an early age. "Hold your head up high." When it comes to the ways in which the body is a metaphor for how we live our lives, this may be one instance where "pulling yourself up by the bootstraps" is not helpful. Lifting the chest and the chin upward not only causes tension in your body but could potentially be related to other kinds of tensions in your life.

It takes practice and patience to get used to the new feelings that come with letting the head balance on top of the spine. Relaxing your belly helps relax the neck, which helps release tension at the atlanto-occipital joint. Part II will give specific guidelines for finding just where your head's neutral position can be found. For many people, this comes as a great relief.

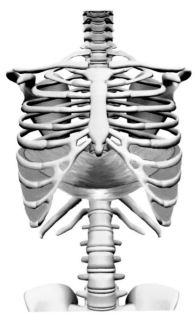

Inhale

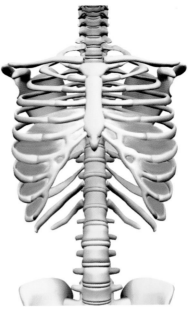

Exhale

On inhalation, the diaphragm flattens down and outward as it contracts into the abdominal cavity. It creates negative air space in the lungs so that air gets pulled into them, much like the action of a piston in an engine. This action kneads the organs of digestion and elimination, gently pressing and squeezing them with each inhalation and assisting in their efficient functioning. When we are in the habit of breathing into the upper chest and not the lower back or abdomen, our organs miss out on this necessary massage. Diaphragmatic breathing is tied into the parasympathetic nervous system and sends a signal that all is well and we can rest in a state of calm.

The diaphragm relaxes into its dome shape on exhalation. Slouching when we sit or stand as well as actively lifting up our chest and rib cage impinges on the diaphragm, tightening the muscle fibers and attachments and binding them up with tension. This restricts the diaphragm's natural, easy movement and signals the sympathetic nervous system that all may not be well. This is yet one more way that natural alignment has a profound effect on our overall health and well-being.

It is impossible to study one large system, such as the respiratory system, completely by itself. The body is like a giant symphony orchestra with an almost infinite number of instruments, all of which are interconnected and contribute to the music that it produces. In terms of the body, none of the systems ever plays solo. Each is dependent upon and affected by another. The autonomic nervous system, charged with maintaining a state of equilibrium and homeostasis in all bodily systems and functions, takes its cues from the quality of the breath and tension of the muscles. Likewise, signals from the nervous system trigger a response in the muscles and the respiratory system.

No muscles are more important in this neuromuscular interchange than those muscles located in the abdomen, the area of the body's center of gravity—the viscera, the core, our "guts." Included among these muscles are the diaphragm, *rectus abdominis, transversus abdominis* and the psoas muscles. All four of these muscle groups help determine whether the parasympathetic or sympathetic nervous system is in charge at any given time. The alignment of our bones can determine whether these muscles are free to relax or not.

Abdominal core strength is a natural byproduct of living in an aligned way. Artificially strengthening our abdominal muscles shortens the distance between the *pubic symphysis* and the sternum, leading to contraction and shortening of the spine. Because of the restriction this causes to the diaphragm, this ultimately affects our overall health as well as how we age.

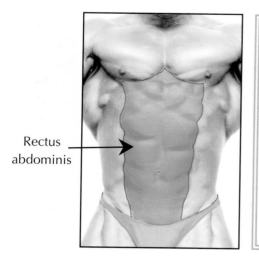

Rectus
abdominis

Our cultural obsession with having firm abdominals binds up the diaphragm and creates stress for our entire system. The sympathetic fight-or-flight response is turned on in a low-grade, chronic state. Chances are we don't even recognize that this is happening since our regular state of tension has become our norm and we no longer know what it feels like to be fully and naturally relaxed.

It is likely that you think of your abdominal muscles as being located in the front of the body. In fact, your deepest layer of abdominal muscles, the *transversus abdominis,* wrap around the lower torso much like a built-in corset, helping to stabilize your structure. Most muscles move bones, but the "trans ab" muscle is a support muscle that is naturally toned and elastic simply by virtue of fulfilling its important role.

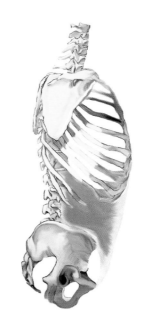

This muscle is unable to fulfill this role, however, when the *rectus abdominis,* the more superficial abdominal muscle that runs up and down the front of the abdomen, is too tightly contracted. Exercises designed to firm up the abs and flatten the belly only serve to compound the problem, causing a chronic shortening within the spine. The problems caused by the over-development of the rectus muscle can be serious after a time. This concept can be difficult to accept; it runs counter to almost everything we currently believe about health and fitness. Indeed, firm abs are at the heart of our current notion of fitness.

Tightening of the *rectus abdominis* muscle draws the *pubis symphysis* upward, causing the pelvis to tuck under. This is what happens when we "suck and tuck." As the sit bones are pulled downward toward the back of the knees, the hamstring muscles become shortened. Shortened hamstrings contribute to a backward tilt of the pelvis, which interferes with the necessary angle of the sacral platform to support the spine. We then often attempt to counteract the ensuing collapse along the spine above by lifting the chest, thus tensing throughout the torso and neck and placing stress on the nervous system.

The secret to natural, upright carriage is abdominal muscles that are relaxed and elastic and allow our bones to align easily. Tension in abdominal muscles often comes about from the way we sit and stand and bend and causes the spine to compress and be unnaturally distorted. This is a primary cause of our getting shorter as we age.

So As the Psoas, So Is the Pelvis

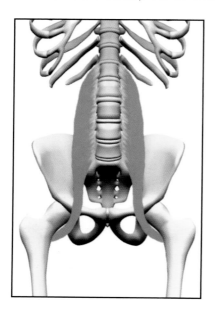

A relaxed psoas is vital to free movement of the pelvis, hips, legs, spine and diaphragm. It provides elastic support for uprightness in addition to creating the right conditions for soft, natural breathing, an optimally extended spine and an engaged parasympathetic nervous system (relaxation response).

Many people are unaware of one of the most important muscles they have, the psoas (pronounced so-as). Located deep within the torso behind the abdominal organs, the psoas joins the trunk to the legs, passing across the front of the pelvis and hip joint and attaching to the inside of the femur. The psoas plays a crucial role in maintaining natural uprightness and in determining the position of the pelvis.

When the skeleton is aligned, the psoas can be free and elastic, performing its multiple roles as hip flexor, guy wire, pelvic stabilizer and support hammock for abdominal organs. When skeletal support is missing, the psoas becomes tight and clenched, causing tension deep at its core. This tension can translate into back and hip pain as well as being linked to feelings of anxiety and emotional discomfort.

Learning to sense one's psoas is the first step in being able to release it from holding tension. Core strength is not synonymous with core tightness. Tightness at the core closes off and prevents the flow of easy movement, which prevents the dynamic support of aligned bones and free movement of energy so necessary to healthy living.

Few muscles are as involved in multitasking as the psoas, which counterbalances at least four different muscles: the *rectus abdominis, erector spinea, obturators* and *transversospinalis*. It also merges with the *iliacus* muscle. Paradoxically, the psoas can produce two opposite effects on the movement of the lumbar spine. It can tighten in one way to tilt the pelvis forward, creating a deeper curve in the lumbar spine

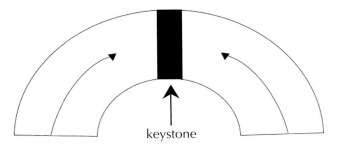

keystone

It is no wonder that creative evolution settled on arches for support. Arches are used in architecture and found throughout nature for good reason.

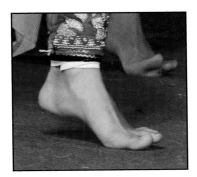 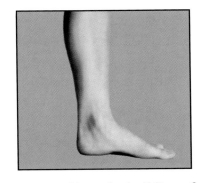

Throughout history, arches have been incorporated into the building of bridges, cathedrals and temples because of the strength of this design. There are instances where the keystone at the top of the arch is not mortared but held in place by the two halves of the arch rising up to meet and hold the keystone in place with a pressure that has withstood the passage of centuries. Weight that is distributed evenly from above serves to increase the pressure of the two halves coming together, thus increasing their strength as well.

When arches of the feet are well developed, they allow for flexibility and mobility of the feet. The muscles that are required to raise up the arches are the same muscles that work to stabilize the ankle and knee joints. The importance of having a good foundation is much more important in a human body than in a building. Human bodies have far more complex requirements than buildings that stand unmoving. Human bodies walk and bend, dance and carry, all of which require an aligned foundation as well as a shifting center of gravity that allows for both stability and easy, fluid movement.

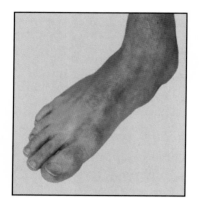 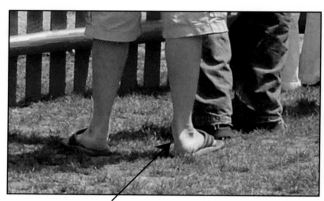

Sheer force pushing ankle inward

Feet like these tend to act like flippers that slap the ground when one walks. Without arches, the feet are unable to provide the body with the shock-absorbing qualities that healthy feet are designed to do. The toes are uninvolved and are of little help in walking.

"Fallen" arches such as the ones seen in these photos contribute to a long list of problems that can develop as a result of faulty support of the foundation. With these arches, the ankle drops inward and the leg bones fall off the top of the ankle platform. This causes a sheer force upon the ankle, which is unstable and prone to being easily twisted and sprained. The knees and hips are also vulnerable when they lack support from below. Muscles of the leg are then torqued and misshapen. This chronic shortening of the muscle fibers begins the body's long, slow descent from being extended and upright. Poor arches make it virtually impossible for the feet to be aligned with the rest of the body.

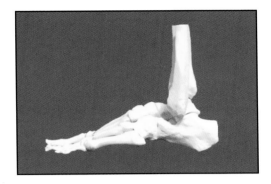

The 26 bones in each foot are arranged in a precise and complex relationship with each other as well as the lower leg bones (tibia and fibula). In a healthy foot, a well-defined and flexible arch is reflected in the height of the top of the foot. The body's weight is distributed primarily on the large, thick heel bone, and the toes connect to the ground or floor to aid with balance.

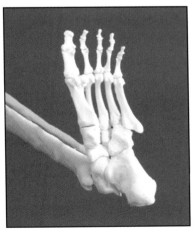
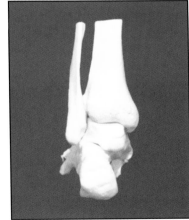

The bones under the ball of the foot are delicate and birdlike, not designed to carry the weight of the body. Most of the weight is intended to come down through the legs and be sent into the dense, bulky heel bone that is perfectly designed to catch weight. Many people with foot problems find relief when they learn how to stand on aligned feet with aligned bones above.

A misaligned foot creates a whole host of problems in the body that stands above it. Without the support of the arches and strong, aligned ankles, problems can occur in the knees, hips, back, shoulders and even neck.

In some populations in the world, especially where people go barefoot much of the time, feet rarely lose the innate qualities of lifted arches and actively working toes. The feet maintain a crescent, or kidney bean, shape, clearly visible in the bottom of the feet pictured on the right.

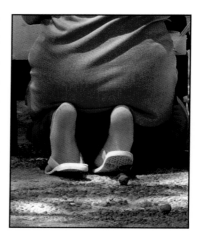

Millions of people the world over walk into old age on strong, healthy feet while developing few modern foot problems such as bunions, hammer toes, heel spurs and plantar fasciitis. The two pairs of feet below belong to a 90-year-old man and his 86-year-old wife. They still work barefoot everyday in the rice paddy behind their house and have rarely worn shoes during their lives. Their feet are remarkable in how much they resemble the feet of young children.

The feet pictured to the right are 103 years old. They helped this woman carry river rocks on her head for several decades. They now help her assist with the daily care of her great-grandson.

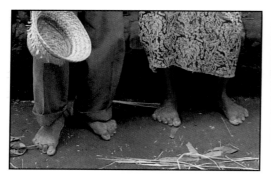

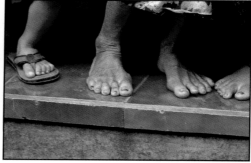

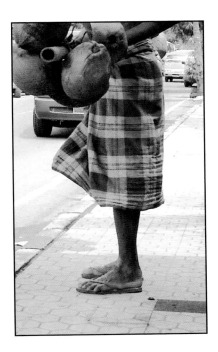 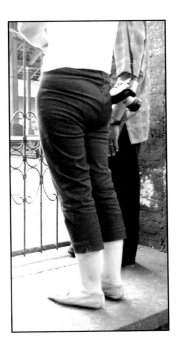

   The alignment of the feet is reflected in the relationship of the legs and pelvis and vice versa. The woman on the left has ankles that drop inward, collapsing her arches and causing her weight to land on the inside of her feet. The fact that her pelvis is tucked under and thrust forward of her ankles means that the weight of her body lands very differently on her feet than the weight lands on the man's feet shown at the right, where it is evenly distributed through a neutral pelvis and leg bones that are vertical. This man's weight comes down through the arches and is passed onto the outside of the heel. The woman on the left already complains of problems in her feet and lower back although she is only in her late 30s. It's not surprising that the man on the right reports no pain even though he is in his mid-70s.

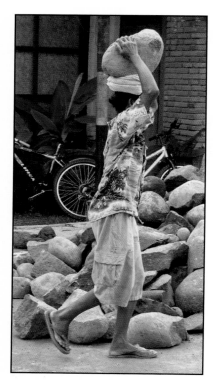

"As above, so below" is an apt expression in describing the relationship between structural alignment and the condition of one's feet. The inverse of this also can be true.

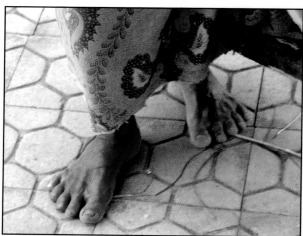

The Scoop on Feet

Healthy feet engage with the ground on which they stand. They serve the body for many decades, and their strength, flexibility and alignment is reflected in the health of the body that stands above them.

The secret to this woman's success is good arch support—not the kind that comes with expensive sports shoes but her own built-in arches. Her feet and legs work so well that they support the pelvis, spine, rib cage and skull in a balanced relationship that allows her to carry rocks like this all day, every day (even on pavement!), and still be smiling at the end of the day.

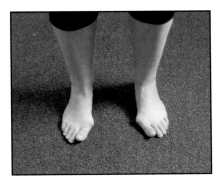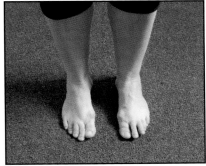

It takes many years for young healthy feet to become misshapen and distorted in the way that these feet are. Notice the prominent bunions and how the ankles fall inward, collapsing the arches and misplacing the leg bones. These feet provide little support for the body that stands above them. They are also prone to pain and injury. Usually, this kind of distortion in the feet is reflected by other distortions in the skeletal structure of the rest of the body.

Less than a minute later, the same feet look like this! This is accomplished through a simple technique called a foot scoop that gently and painlessly rearranges the bones of the feet. Notice how the bunions have all but disappeared, the ankles are realigned to the midline and the arches and tops of the feet have lifted up. While this is no quick fix and the exercises to do it must be repeated regularly until real change occurs from the inside out, almost anyone can learn, with patient practice, to return the feet to their natural, strong alignment and provide the body with the support that it requires. We'll revisit our feet again in Part II and learn ways to bring them back to their natural state.

Chapter Eight
Pregnant with Possibilities
one of which is being comfortable

Pregnancy is a time of great change; a woman's body swells with the growth of life within. It is a time that can present a woman with new challenges, especially when it comes to finding ease and comfort in her body during those last few months of pregnancy. It is not uncommon for expectant mothers to experience back pain, sciatica, heartburn, swollen ankles and insomnia to one degree or another. For some women, these problems can be particularly difficult.

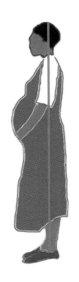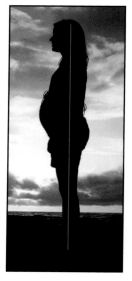

Most women don't realize that many of these problems can be alleviated, at least in part, by knowing how to apply principles of natural alignment. Pregnancy and childbirth are as natural to humans as to all species. It is easy to forget this in the modern world of scheduled caesarean deliveries, fetal-heart monitors, epidurals, fluorescent-lit nurseries and baby bottles. Babies are more likely to thrive when they are born to a mother who is comfortable and relaxed with what is happening to her and who takes care of herself. Chances are good that a woman who is relaxed and comfortable during her pregnancy will be more likely to have an uncomplicated delivery and move into motherhood with greater ease. Among other things, this requires self-awareness and natural structural alignment. Few occasions offer a woman a greater opportunity to turn her attention inward as she shares the months of her pregnancy with the small being growing inside of her.

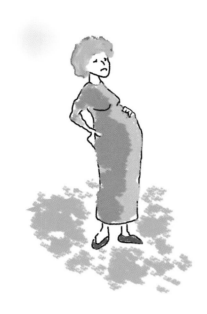

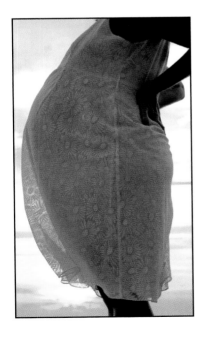

As the baby grows inside the uterus, the weight that is added onto the front of the mother-to-be has the potential to throw her off balance. The majority of pregnant women today, having a higher center of gravity and an out of aligned position to begin with, are required to lean backwards above the waist. This causes the spine to be compressed and puts tremendous stress on the lower back. Not only can this cause back pain, it has the potential to reduce the easy flow of blood, lymph and other fluids that are not only important for the mother's health and comfort but for the baby's as well. Fortunately, a soon-to-be mother can learn how to counteract this tendency by applying basic principles of alignment that may save her back and allow her to have a far more enjoyable pregnancy.

Not only is the back put at risk by the typical pregnant stance, but internal organs that are already crowded by the growing fetus can become even more compressed by faulty posture. This can lead to a whole host of digestive problems, shortness of breath and fatigue. A pregnant woman can learn how to call upon her inherent skeletal support to do the work of holding her up in a way that is comfortable and gives relief from many of the most common problems women experience, especially during the most challenging last months of pregnancy.

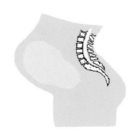

Pregnancy lordosis

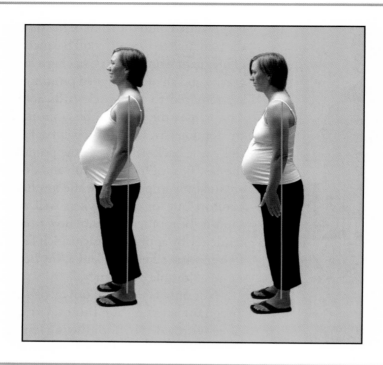

Here we see the hazards of standing out of alignment for a woman who is in the last months of pregnancy. In the photo on the left, most of this mother-to-be's body is displaced forward of the axis, causing the legs to lose their ability to fully support her. Excessive arching of the lower back (lordosis) and an opposite rounding of the upper back (kyphosis) can be the cause of back pain, restricted blood flow and impingement of the diaphragm's ability to function efficiently.

Rather than the baby fitting compactly into the womb (uterus) and being held in place from below by lower belly muscle fibers that serve as a hammock (as seen in the photo on the right), the muscle fibers are askew and the position of the baby is pushed out and forward. We can only guess at the effect this sometimes has, not only on the comfort of the mother during pregnancy but on the baby, the process of delivery and the mother's return to her normal state after the baby is born.

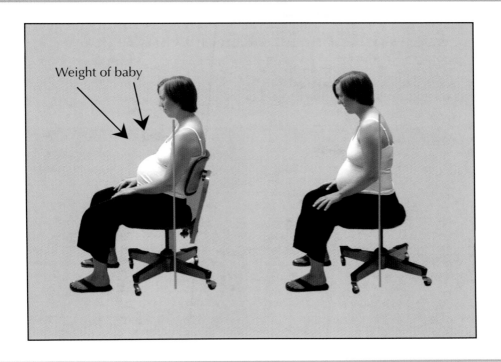

Weight of baby

Sitting in a natural position becomes doubly important for the woman who carries an almost full-term baby in her belly. When she sits without the direct support of her sit bones but instead, with her pelvis tilted backward (photo on left), her torso collapses throughout. Gravity bears downward, pushing the weight of the fetus, placenta and amniotic fluids onto this mother's internal organs. Breathing is restricted, and the diaphragm gets pinched and crowded in this position. It is not difficult to understand why pregnant women complain so often of back pain, heartburn, constipation, fluid retention and shortness of breath.

The mother-to-be who sits on her sit bones and lets her spine support her torso is far less likely to experience these difficulties. It is not difficult to see why since the baby fits neatly and is supported from below by the cross fibers of the *transverses abdominus* and the oblique muscles, rather than the fetus bearing down from above. Sitting this way is good practice for keeping the floor of the pelvis open and relaxed, which can be an important detail during the birthing of the baby.

Knowing how to sit, stand and bend is important for everyone but especially so for the woman who is moving for two. By taking her cue from toddlers who demonstrate how to move in an easy and natural way, she will greatly enhance her ability to enjoy her time being pregnant. Knowing which comfortable positions she can take for sleeping and resting will provide her with ways to practice the important art of relaxing in preparation for the big event of delivery.

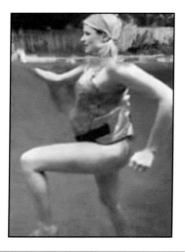

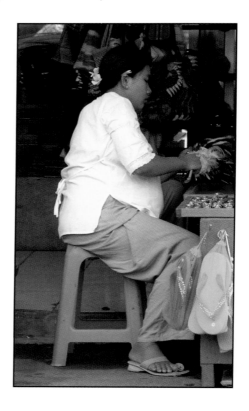

A laboring woman's ability to relax greatly increases her chances for having a natural birth, good for both her and her baby.

Preparation for labor and delivery is greatly enhanced by knowing how to sit and squat in natural ways, how to release the pelvic floor and how to give in to gravity as the baby moves through the birth canal. Any exercises done during pregnancy should adhere to the basic principles of natural alignment and should emphasize relaxing and letting go. Being able to breathe naturally helps the mother to relax and counters tendencies to tense the body during contractions. This aids in the process of the dilation of the cervix and keeps the mother from becoming fatigued before the time arrives for her to push.

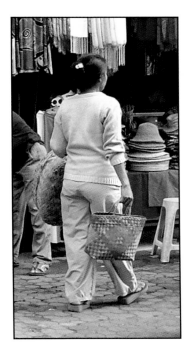 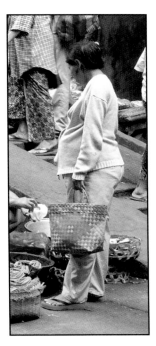 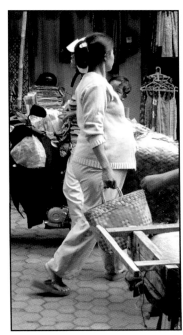

Pregnancy appears to come easily to this young woman who has lived in a naturally aligned body her entire life. Adjusting to the new demands of pregnancy are not difficult. Without ever having to think about it, she knows that her bones will hold her up and thus does not have to throw her upper body behind her natural center in order to compensate for the added weight.

It is difficult to tell from behind that this woman is pregnant, so relaxed and easy is her stature.

Viewed from the side, this woman is seen to be far along in her pregnancy. A return to normal after the baby's birth will probably be accelerated by the ease with which she moved through the pregnancy.

Learning to pay attention to how a new mother inhabits her body gets the mind and body working together to let go of muscular tension and relieve discomfort. It also prepares her to tune in to what is going on under her skin. A very important person is sharing her internal environment. As the mother turns her attention inward, focusing on her breath and relaxing all tension as it arises, she will feel a connection with her baby and a growing confidence in her new role as its mother.

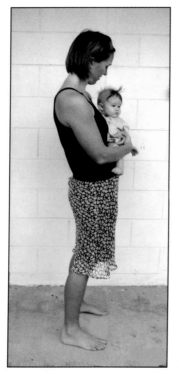 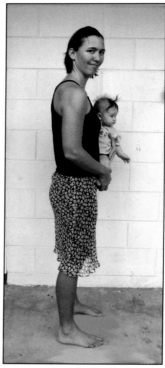

Once the baby is in its mother's arms, many other challenges arise, not the least of which is how to comfortably lift and carry the child who was once carried inside. Breastfeeding, while nourishing the baby like nothing else, can also be less than nourishing for the new mother if her back and neck are aching and tense. Knowing how to place her bones while holding, carrying and lifting the baby will greatly enhance the experience for mother and baby alike.

Chapter Nine
Our Children in Peril
a looming health crisis?

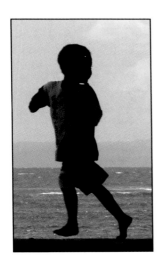 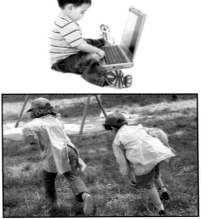 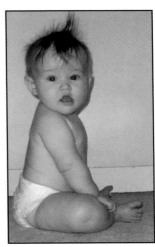

Babies come into the world with very little muscle strength and no understanding of how to sit, crawl, stand or walk. Within the first 12 to 18 months of their lives, almost all of them teach themselves how to do these things. First by lifting and turning their heads, then by kicking their legs and pushing their arms, they gradually develop the coordination, strength and balance required to get themselves from a horizontal to a vertical position. At this point, it appears that muscle strength is at least matched by an ability to balance the skeletal bones in relationship to each other. In order for a child to maintain relaxed alignment in the years ahead, this relationship must continue. Like all mammal babies, human children have a great capacity for playfulness. Child's play is serious business, wherein babies diligently apply themselves, among other things, to the task of mastering the art of movement.

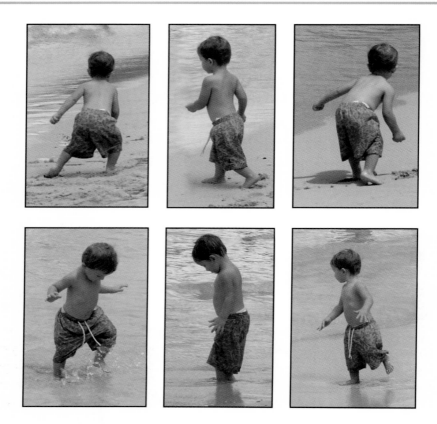

This little boy is a master of natural movement. His playfulness at the beach models how the human body is designed to work with efficiency, comfort and ease. Every move he makes maintains the integrity of his spine's alignment, so it is possible for him to be both relaxed and physically active at the same time. No unnecessary muscular tension is called into play; only that required to move the bones by bending at the appropriate joints. Anyone wanting to relearn how to move naturally could take lessons from this child as well as almost all children at this age.

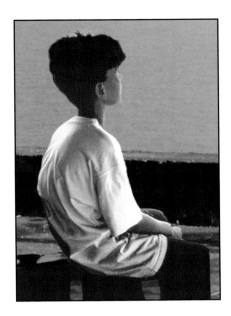 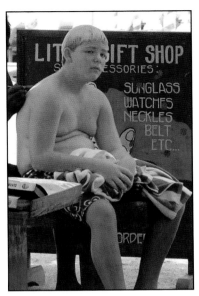

These two boys, who at one time almost certainly looked and moved like the toddler on the previous page, have somehow become so collapsed away from the center of alignment that they actually sit on their sacrum and tailbone (coccyx) rather than the sit bones *(ischial tuberosities)*. This is a serious situation that developed over a period of very few years. This is the epidemic that children are facing all over the world. It causes their vital organs to be compressed to the point where functions relating to respiration, digestion, assimilation of nutrients and elimination of waste are bound to be affected. In addition, the flow of blood through veins and arteries is likely to be constricted, the configuration of many muscle fibers is distorted and the range of motion in their joints is limited by bones that are jammed together.

The spines of these two boys are severely deformed in this position, which puts pressure on the spinal cord and is likely to put the nervous systems under assault. Their bones are still growing, and the way their weight is distributed through their bones could well affect the way their bones grow. Most parents and teachers are essentially unaware of the seriousness of this problem—and if they are, unsure what to do about it—making it unlikely that these boys are going to become educated or supported in making a change.

While research has not addressed the relationship between natural alignment and health, it is hard to imagine that these boys' health would not be affected by their habitual patterns of use—or misuse.

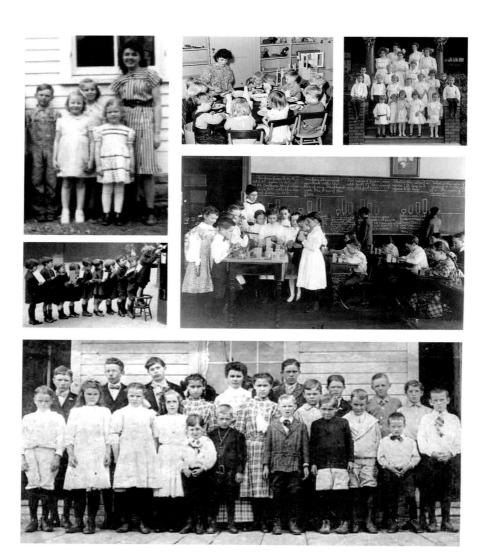

A look at class photos "then" and "now" is very revealing. Almost every child in these photographs is standing on two straight legs or sitting directly on sit bones. Their bodies are well supported by aligned skeletons, their clothes drape without excessive wrinkling, and their hems are level. They are formal but not stiff.

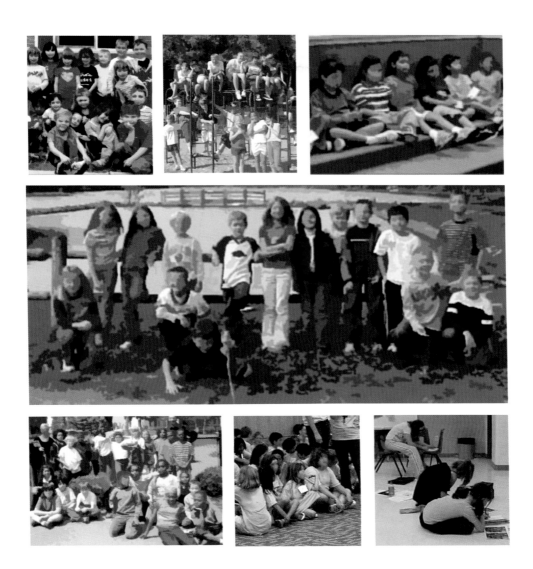

By contrast, few of these children remember what it means to live as natural human beings. This is unfortunate because even at this young age, many of them are already suffering from pain and tension. Physical activity is no longer the playful pastime that it once was for many of them; their bodies do not move with the same ease and freedom they did only a few years ago when they were toddlers. As they forget how to sit, stand or move in ways that are natural, they will never return to where they started unless they re-learn what to do and commit to applied practice.

The contrast between still-aligned and no-longer-aligned children is not only evident between years past and the present but between children here in the United States and children who live in some other places in the world.

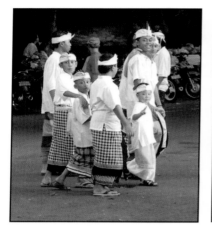 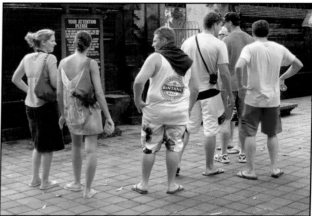

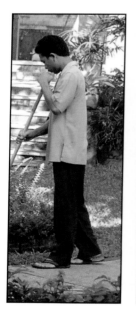 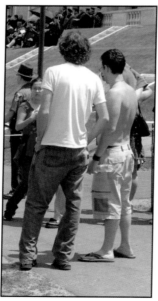

A relaxed, flowing quality is evident among those young people who live in naturally aligned bodies. Their clothing hangs smoothly and evenly, giving them a graceful, flowing appearance that matches the symmetry of the skeletons that support them. Young people who are not aligned often take on a variety of shapes, none of which are natural. They may shift their weight back and forth between one leg and the other while standing, display over-development of certain muscles (most typically across the shoulders) and wear clothing that is bunched and wrinkled.

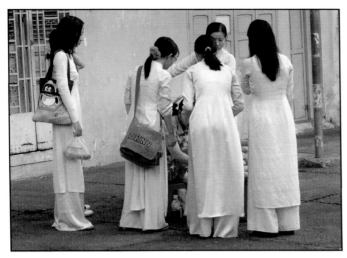
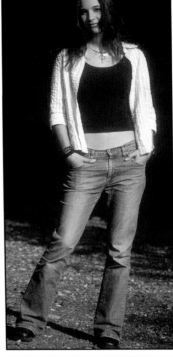
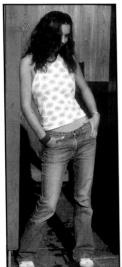
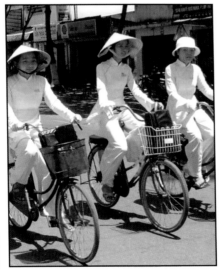
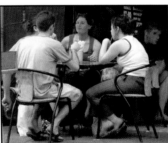

While there is an obvious difference in dress styles, these are cultural and generally irrelevant to what is actually going on under the clothing. When looking at the aligned teenagers, it is obvious that their bodies organize themselves around the central axis, that their spines are neither collapsed nor hyper-extended and arched, that their legs are positioned to hold them up. Such is the case whether they are standing or sitting, and in both instances, reveal that same, relaxed quality of being.

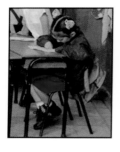 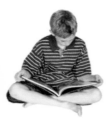 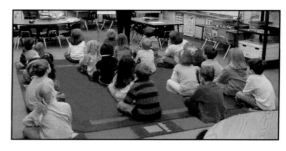

Many things contribute to the problem of poor posture—certain types of strollers, car seats, baby carriers, etc., that babies are put into from an early age as well as the kinds of desk chairs commonly used in classrooms. All of these often place the pelvis in a backward tilt, a position that is often held for hours every day. Thus begins the habitual patterns of use that become set into muscle fibers and draw children away from inhabiting their bodies in a natural way. These patterns are repeated again and again until they dictate how most children use their bodies in everything they do and, eventually, how they will age in the years to come.

Postural habits adopted by children in the early years of schooling are likely to remain with them throughout their lives. Just what are the effects of chronic distortion of the spine on children's nervous systems? Is it possible that a relationship exists between how we sit and how we learn? Or how we feel? Or how we relate to others and events in our environment? Are there certain postural patterns that are common to children who struggle with particular types of learning disabilities? Depression? Autism? Maybe not, but are we doing a disservice to our children by dismissing these questions without first examining them?

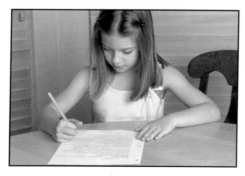 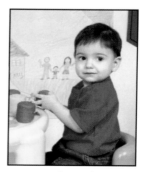

Aligned   Aligned

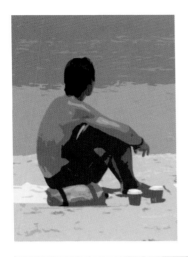
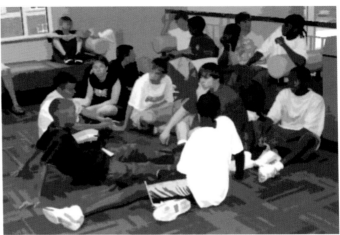
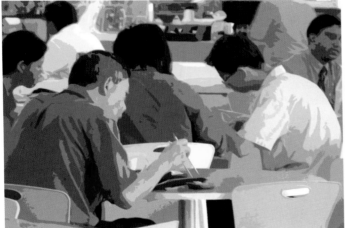
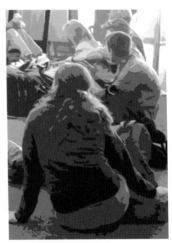

By the time children reach their teens and become young adults, these patterns and habits are so deeply embedded into their physical being that it is all but impossible for them to revert to what is natural. Nothing less than educating them about the situation, along with clear instructions and continuous positive reinforcement, can encourage them to redirect these habits. It is far easier for parents and teachers to help children reverse these habits at a much younger age. It is also far easier to address this situation when children are still young enough to be inhabiting their bodies according to its design. Then, it is only a matter of creating the conditions that interfere as little as possible with what is natural and support them in remaining aligned and relaxed.

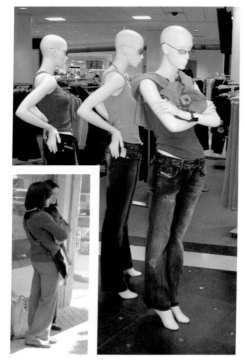

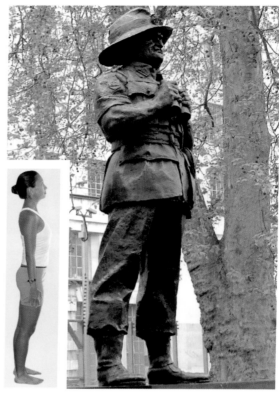

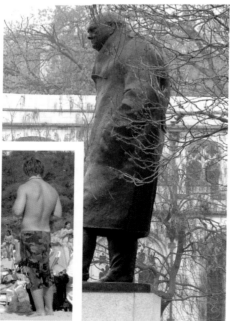

One way we can support our children in remaining natural is in examining the part that certain role models or pop idols play and the messages that we regularly put before them. While there is no need to stop honoring or looking up to these people, there may be some value in acknowledging that some of our cultural icons, both past and present, as great as we may believe they are, do not demonstrate the good posture that comes with relaxed, natural alignment. Over time, as our awareness of what natural alignment is and how important it is to our health and wellbeing, it may be that our icons themselves will begin to reflect the changes happening within us.

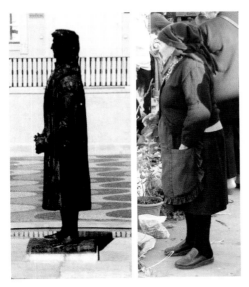

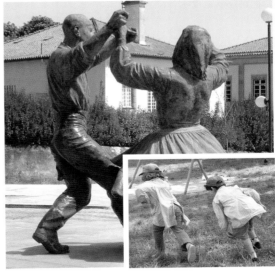

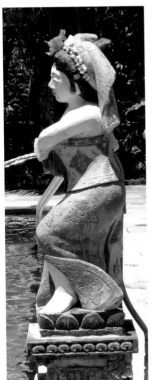

In some places in the world different examples predominate. Not surprisingly, a greater number of people in these places appear to reflect the natural alignment of the statues and icons in their environment.

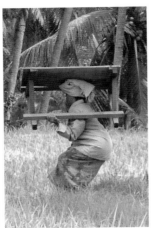

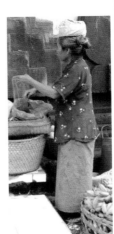

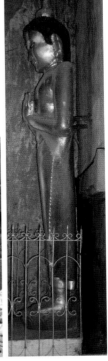

Playtime Reinvented

Once upon a time, playtime consisted of running, jumping, skipping and climbing in the backyard or neighborhood park or in nearby woodlands. Young children played kick-the-can and tag in loosely organized neighborhood groups. Physical activity was a typical pastime. Today, they are just as likely to be sitting in front of a television or a computer screen. The percentage of overweight six-to-eleven-year-olds has more than tripled in the last 30 years. Fewer and fewer children walk or ride bicycles to school, often driven by parents 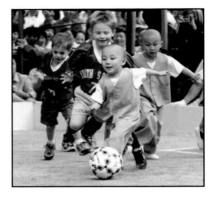 who are on their way to work. While many children are going the way of a more sedentary lifestyle, many others are specializing in particular sports at younger ages. Participating in sports can be an important activity for many children, rich with an array of benefits, and certainly an appealing alternative to the couch-potato syndrome some of their friends have opted for instead.

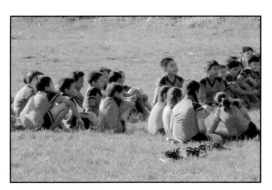 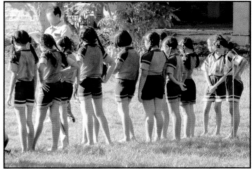

Children are likely to benefit from playing sports when their bodies are natural and their movements are free, as with the young boys pictured above. If they are supported through other activities and cultural influences to continue to move according to their bodies' design, they will be far less likely to experience injuries. The young girls pictured below are at a great disadvantage and are more likely candidates for injury and pain because so few of their bodies still move in free-flowing natural ways. The girl standing at the far right appears to be a striking exception.

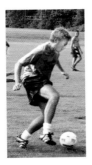
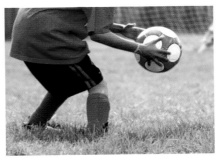
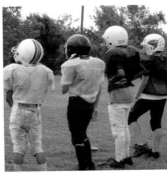
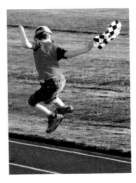

Children whose skeletons are misaligned and whose muscles must work under strain at all times are ill-equipped to participate in sports because they are put at great risk of suffering injuries. The rate of injuries among children that doctors are treating is growing at a disturbing rate, yet the condition that children's bodies are in when they first begin to play a sport is rarely considered to be a factor. Children's bodies are still developing, and some of these injuries have serious implications for the future, such as leading to arthritis and repeated surgeries.

The children pictured here are representative of many children today whose bodies no longer move easily and naturally. (The boy jumping at far right above still demonstrates natural, efficient movement). The constant repetition of certain movements when muscles are working in an unnatural way to begin with is brutal to these children's joints, which is where many of their problems appear—elbows, knees, ankles and hips. Many sports injuries affect ligaments, which connect bone to bone at the joints, and can be particularly problematic. Repair of the anterior cruciate ligament (ACL) that helps hold the knee together is commonplace in children today, whereas 20 years ago it was rare for someone under age 15 to have this surgery. Pediatric orthopedic surgery is a relatively new specialty that has grown up in response to the increasing number of youthful injuries.

Techno-Babies

Some children spend many hours a day, their spines curled and collapsed, in front of televisions and computer screens. The proliferation of video games that hold a special appeal to many children only compounds the problem. Added to that is the fact that the chairs they sit in both at home and at school and the height of the screen and keyboard often force them to sit in ways that reinforce poor habits of use.

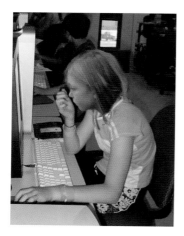
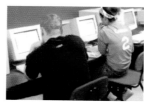
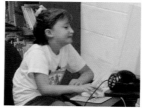
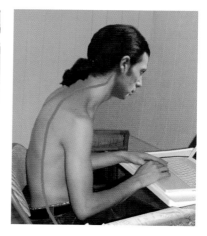

These children pictured below are fortunate to be supported by erect spines. If they maintain this aligned, relaxed posture while at the computer, their use of the computer will be far less physically problematic.

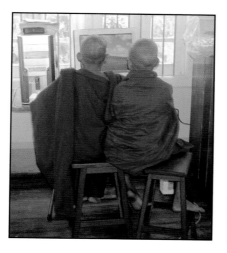
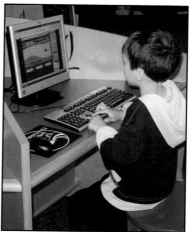

The more we understand how our bodies are designed to work, the more tools we have to work with in implementing changes in the way we exercise and move in general. This can still be quite challenging because it requires such a wholesale paradigm shift in how the body is inhabited, dramatically changing our relationship with a body that we've been somewhat disconnected from for much of our lives. This change is a gradual process that occurs over time, building slowly on itself from the inside out. The very foundation of this process lies in a willingness to be mindful and aware of ourselves as much of the time as possible. Without an interest in developing this capacity, this kind of deep, organic change cannot take place. If we can accept that aligned, balanced posture is beautiful in its natural form, we no longer need to be driven to exercise simply for the sake of a culturally-imposed standard of appearance and can relax into accepting our own "ideal" body.

> "A person who has been holding his chest high...feels when first told to disregard his chest in accordance with better mechanical adjustment, that he is losing some of his moral force by so doing...Effective responses to new sensations and better coordinated action will bring about new habits, or new patterns of posture, which in time will feel comfortable."
> —Mabel Todd, *The Thinking Body,* 1937

The meaning of true health is marked by a body composition that is ideal to the natural individual, by strength and flexibility that results from an interplay of bones, muscles and connective tissue working together naturally, by efficient cardio-respiratory function, by free range of motion of all joints, agility, balance, coordination and stamina. Most important to good health is free flow of life energy and an ongoing quality of relaxation, even while under various types of stress. When we explore these qualities more closely, it becomes apparent that each one of them relates to and is affected in some way by skeletal alignment.

The meaning of fitness, on the other hand, is less clear. Dictionaries expose the confusion of linguists, with some defining fitness as possessing a quality of overall health, while others emphasize a quality of developed strength through exercise. Overall, fitness today has evolved into being more about performance, a measurement of one's functional capacity to accomplish certain goals. Although health reflects an absence of disease, this meaning of fitness does not necessarily reflect an absence of disease, nor does it suggest anything about the actual condition of overall health. Health is an underlying quality of the entire organism, from the condition of the cardiovascular system and the elasticity of the diaphragm to the ability to relax.

Fitness, in terms of its current cultural meaning, dwells more at the surface, where it can be readily observed through muscles that have a pronounced shape. Today, one would probably not use the word "fit" to describe someone with soft, pliable muscles, even if this person happened to possess better overall health than someone with tremendously developed muscles, who would be far more likely to be described as "fit."

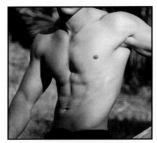

Distorted spine and contracted diaphragm

Health suggests a heart that is strong, with blood flowing freely through unrestricted blood vessels, breathing that is smooth and efficient, a nervous system that regularly restores itself in the parasympathetic mode and an overall condition of the body that is not likely to succumb to disease. Fitness promises none of these things. Fitness, at least by the most common definition, does not require that the nervous systems be in a healthy condition. Indeed, exercise may contribute to people feeling less stressed and more relaxed. Both stress and an inability to fully relax can become more deeply-established in a body that displays a high level of fitness, where muscles are regularly shortened and tight, the spine and spinal cord are repeatedly compressed and distorted, and the diaphragm's ability to breathe efficiently is restricted.

A Gallery of Bona-Fide Fitness

If we were to refine the meaning of fitness to include an underlying quality of health made possible by:

1) an optimally extended spine
2) elastic muscles with minimal stored-up tension
3) open, free-moving joints
4) relaxed, natural breathing
5) an ability to fully and deeply relax

This is what true fitness would look like.

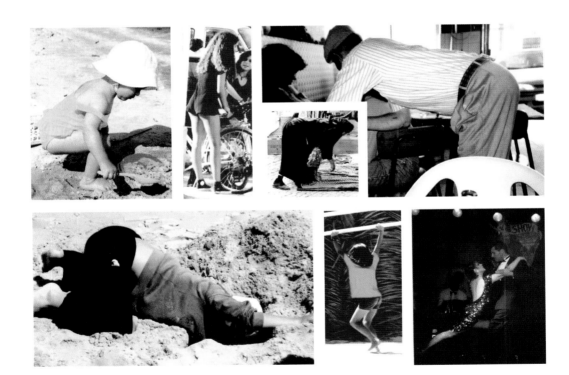

Actively stretching muscles has grown in popularity in recent years. Stretching is typically understood as being necessary for relieving stiffness, maintaining flexibility, avoiding compression of joints and enhancing free movement. Unfortunately, the kind of flexibility that is gained from active stretching must be repeated on a regular basis. Natural flexibility is always available as a by-product of living in a body that is structurally aligned. With the bones of the body positioned in a natural relationship to each other, muscles simply are relaxed and free of tension and, therefore, inherently flexible.

This concept can be difficult to accept. One reason is that it runs counter to many messages that are regularly repeated about the benefits of stretching. Another reason is that stretching feels so good. Lengthening muscle fibers through stretching releases tension that has been stored up in tense, tight muscles, providing a sense of relief and an enhanced ability to relax—for a time. This may be one of the reasons that stretching programs of all sorts are so popular today, particularly since so many people live in bodies that are no longer naturally aligned. Misaligned bones cause tension to be stored in chronically contracted muscle fibers and fascial webbing. Stretching works well as a short-term remedy for this tension, but in the long run, it can result in over-stretched ligaments and tendons, hyper-mobility in joints, muscle strains and tears, and a dependence on regular stretching in order to feel good. While some people who consistently work at developing greater flexibility are able to perform remarkable feats, hyper-flexibility is not a prerequisite for living in a healthy body.

> **An aligned and balanced body has no need for either extreme strength or flexibility yet has more than enough of each to function in all activities of daily living. This natural strength and flexibility can be maintained with little effort well into old age.**

Stretching can be beneficial for therapeutic purposes, but only if it is never forced and is practiced in ways that hold to the rules of movement set down by our body's design. Stretching is the active pulling of the ends of muscle fibers away from each other. It is far more beneficial, once the bones are aligned, to encourage release and letting go in a muscle than to actively pull or stretch it. In the long run, genuine, lasting flexibility comes about only when the skeleton is naturally aligned, which allows muscles to relax. When bones are not aligned, tension always returns, to be relieved once again through a repetitive cycle of stretching. When we attempt to stretch certain muscles, such as the hamstrings at the back of the thigh (see photos below), we often sacrifice the integrity of the spine's alignment while locking poor patterns of use into place. Natural bending always requires that the pelvis first rotate over the head of the femur (thigh bone) in the same way that babies bend. The release of the hamstrings will simply come about as the body gradually aligns itself over time and begins to move in more natural ways. This approach is different from actively imposing flexibility whereby we encounter resistance that can be a set up for injury and pain. (See "How to Bend" in Part III).

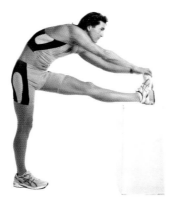
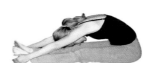

Real flexibility comes about through the capacity of bones to inter-relate by way of mobile joints that are moved by elastic muscles in a natural way. This does not come about by indiscriminate stretching of specific muscles at the expense of the integrity of the spine.

Bend Like a Baby

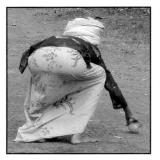
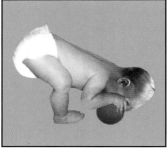
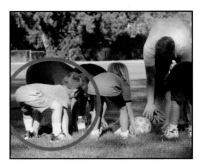

Young children bend by rotating the pelvis over the head of the femur (thigh bone), while bending their knees and bringing their butt up behind them. Their spines remain long and extended. As seen in the photo above, it doesn't take long for many children to lose this understanding, as the coach here has done. Tucking the tailbone under instead of rotating the pelvis over the head of the femur causes unnatural bending along the spine and puts one at risk of injury and pain.

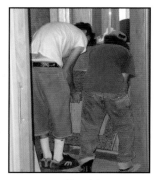
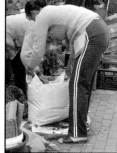
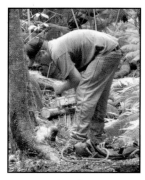

Ouch!   Ouch!   Ouch!

Standing Tall and Firm

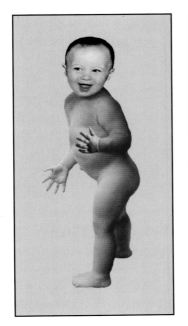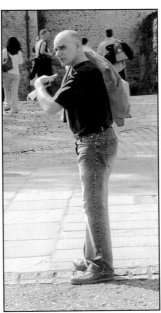

Standing firm means standing on strong legs that give us all the support we need. Without strong legs, the rest of the body must struggle to compensate, fighting against its natural design to hold itself together.

The primary buttock muscle (gluteus maximus) functions as part of the leg. It is the largest muscle in the body, with good reason. It not only works as the primary hip extensor, but it also propels us forward when we walk with aligned bones. The "glutes" also come into play in the process of sitting down, standing up, climbing stairs and bending. For this reason, people with aligned skeletons have well-developed buttock muscles that are full and high up. Buttocks that have a flattened look, or that seem to slide downward, tell a different story, one of retroversion of the pelvis and an unnatural way of moving.

This baby and this man seem worlds apart—one is young and soft, the other large and strong. Yet, in spite of these differences, they also have much in common. They both stand on strong legs that support a pelvis in a neutral position. Each has a relaxed belly, well-developed buttocks and a rib cage that is suspended from its attachments at the back of the spine. Both the baby and the man have long spines that extend all the way through long necks and a well-placed head balanced on top.

Stand Up Straight Means Stand Up Straight

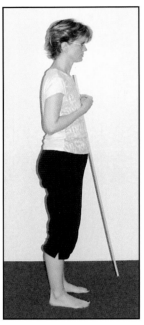

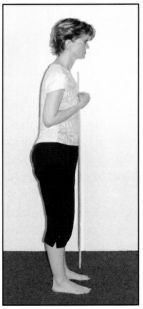

The angle of the breastbone (sternum) reflects the angle of the spine. By holding a dowel against the breastbone you will have a clear indication of whether or not your spine is straight.

The photograph on the top matches what most of us typically equate with standing up straight. Yet the angle of the stick (red line) reveals a backward leaning spine, caused by a backward turning rib cage. Looking more closely, we see that the tailbone is tucked under and the pubis is lifted up, indicating a backward turning pelvis as well. This translates into shortening of the spine and tension in back muscles, especially the lower back (lumbar) area.

It can be discouraging at first to discover that even with a straight spine your head may be positioned further forward than you think it should be (middle photo). Over time, as genuine length comes into the spine, the upper back and cervical vertebrae will lengthen and the head will gradually move back on top of the spine (bottom photo). There is no shortcut for this. Pushing the chest forward to get the head back gives the illusion of uprightness (top photo), but this causes the spine to arch back and leads to serious consequences down the road. For this reason, it is essential to begin from the ground up—feet, legs, pelvis, rib cage, shoulders, neck—each depending on the parts below for the support required for surrounding muscles to relax.

It takes time for the habits and patterns that are stored up in our muscles to remap themselves after all these years. Some changes take days, others months, still others years. All of them are worth it.

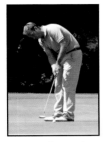 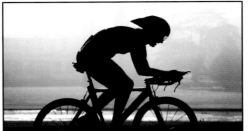 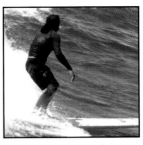

Not aligned   Not aligned   Not aligned

Most sports—from running to basketball to cycling—can put great stress on the body when it must work against its natural design. Many athletes today have far greater muscular power, (occasionally with the help of steroids) than they did just twenty years ago. Many of those who win the competitions do so by relying on forced control and muscular effort. This is not always the case, however. There are many notable examples of top performing athletes (see Endnotes) who engage themselves much of the time in accord with their body's design for movement. While doing so does not make them immune to ever having to suffer pain or injury, anymore than it guarantees them a gold medal or a trophy, it does allow them to accomplish their movements more efficiently, with less reliance on effort and rigid control. Maintaining the integrity of an extended spine is essential to injury-free, pain-free sports activity.

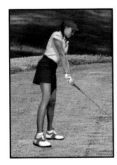 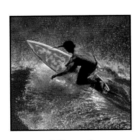 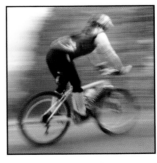

Aligned   Aligned   Aligned

Working In, Not Working Out

Of the many approaches to movement and exercise, the ones that are particularly compatible with natural movement are some of the non-combative martial arts such as QI QONG, TAI CHI and AIKIDO. These modalities were developed during times in history when most people still remained naturally aligned. The movements are slow and place an emphasis on awareness, breathing, movement of energy and the body's alignment. If one is fortunate to already be aligned and relaxed, then these movements serve to reinforce these habits. If one is not aligned, these movements can be helpful in introducing natural patterns of movement into the body when learned from a teacher who understands these concepts.

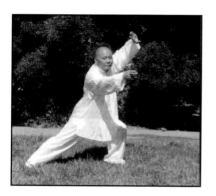 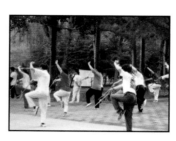 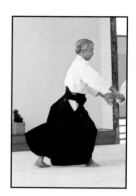

Releasing unskillful habits of use often requires that we slow down, withdraw our fixation on muscular strength, turn our awareness inward and begin to pay attention in a focused way.

Not all people who teach Aikido, Qi Qong or Tai Chi live in aligned bodies themselves. It is important to find a teacher who has been well-trained in traditional techniques and who embodies these principles, not just in the instructions he or she gives in the class but in the way this person stands, walks, bends and sits. This is an important demonstration of the teacher's qualifications.

YOGA is an ancient art and science of living that includes a healthy diet, meditation, living with integrity and the practice of asana, or yoga postures. In the West, yoga primarily focuses on the physical postures and has grown in popularity in recent years, in part because of its tension-releasing features. Many people benefit greatly from the enhanced ability to relax and the increased awareness they often gain from a yoga practice. However, yoga can be problematic if not done in a way that abides by the principles of natural alignment, putting one at risk of strain or injury and entrenching unhelpful habits. Yoga as it is practiced today often emphasizes performance and achievement of goals that can interfere with the deeper benefits to be experienced.

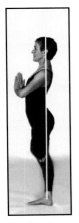
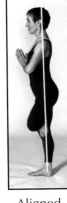
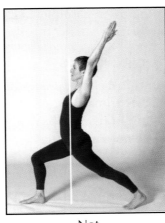
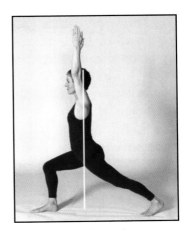

Not aligned   Aligned   Not aligned   Aligned

Jean Couch (above), who has developed "Yoga in Balance," demonstrates yoga postures done both in and out of natural alignment. Yoga postures are often practiced with the body thrust forward of the central axis, unnaturally arching and shortening the spine. Almost all yoga postures can be adapted and practiced in a relaxed way that reinforces natural alignment. It makes sense to suppose that yoga was originally practiced in this aligned way when it was first developed in India thousands of years ago.

Body Works

Those who embark on a gradual process of undoing multiple layers of tension and reorganizing their structure can draw support from a varied palette of bodywork that can lend support by helping to release tension and remap the body. These include hands-on approaches such as massage, Rolfing, chiropractic, trigger point therapy, myofascial release, Zero Balancing and Cranio-Sacral Therapy. Energetic therapies include acupuncture, Reiki, Healing Touch, Therapeutic Touch and Quantum Healing. Re-education and movement approaches to bodywork include Balance, Alexander Technique, Feldenkrais and Aston Patterning. Some of these combine various aspects of touch with movement. There are many others, and, in the hands of a competent practitioner, any one of these can be useful in ways, either large or small, for helping the body release tensions and gradually return to its natural home base.

Three approaches to becoming more naturally aligned will be discussed briefly here because they are especially beneficial and together, they integrate important elements related to this process.

ROLFING, or Structural Integration, is a system of soft tissue manipulation that can achieve remarkable results in helping guide the body toward more natural alignment. Developed by Ida Rolf, its primary focus is on the body's myofascial system of connective tissue and on helping to reorganize the body's relationship to gravity and the central axis. Rolfing, while not an essential ingredient to realigning oneself, can serve as a complementary adjunct for accelerating this process when practiced by an accomplished rolfer with a sensitive touch. In the end, there is nothing that can bring a body back into authentically aligned balance except the directed awareness of the person choosing to change. Rolfing can serve as an important catalyst and support for this change. (See Appendix for further information.)

BALANCE is a complete and effective approach to movement education that provides one with the tools needed for knowing how to live in a naturally aligned and relaxed body. Balance offers very specific and accurate guidelines for how to sit, stand, bend, walk, lift, carry and even sleep in natural, balanced alignment. People discover that they can relieve pain and other problems in many places in their bodies simply by aligning their skeleton to its natural "home base" in all that they do. This approach is built on an examination of the human body's natural design and closely matches what is detailed in this book. Balance gives people concrete tools for putting this information to use in their own lives. The how-to guidelines in Part II are based on the pioneering work of Jean Couch, originator of Balance and founder of the Balance Center. (See Appendix for contact information.)

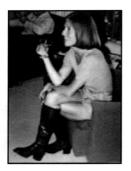

Jean Couch,
Before Balance

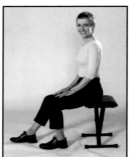

Jean Couch,
After Balance

MINDFULNESS MEDITATION develops inner awareness through a practice of being mindful of your one's present experience. By cultivating an ability to consciously experience the present moment, awareness deepens. This is an ongoing process of investigation in which experience is observed without judgment as it occurs and as one is participating in it. Meditation is enhanced by knowing how to sit in a natural way because energy flows more freely when the body is aligned. Posture affects as well as reflects our state of mind, and meditators find that knowing how to sit in an aligned way can greatly enhance their practice. Among the many benefits to be gained from mindfulness meditation is the ability to focus on the finer details of alignment along with an opportunity to develop greater awareness, an essential ingredient for learning how to consciously and persistently direct one's attention toward home base. (See Sitting to Meditate in Part III.)

Sitting Pretty

One of the first things children teach themselves to do after rolling over is to sit up. In doing this, they don't rely on firm abdominal or back muscles to hold them up—in fact babies are still 'squishy' soft at this stage—but instead discover how to establish a sold seat on their sit bones. Once they've discovered this, their pelvis provides support for a supple extended spine that stacks itself upward with a head balanced delicately on top.

The solid seat is something that all healthy babies figure out for themselves. They are deeply rooted through the sit bones, the floor of the pelvis is soft, not contracted and their muscles, particularly the belly muscles, are comfortably relaxed.

Children who maintain a solid seat throughout childhood are far more likely to enjoy all the benefits of natural strength and easy mobility that will continue in the years ahead. A child who loses this solid seat—something that is happening to more and more children at younger and younger ages—has already embarked on a journey of accelerated aging. (See "How to Sit" Part III).

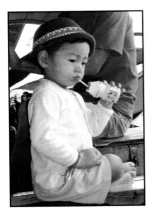 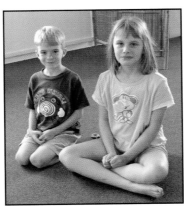 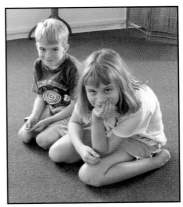

Bracing To Lift, Carry Or Push

When we live in aligned bodies, our deepest core muscles have natural tone and firmness without ongoing contraction. As the most superficial abdominal muscles let go of chronic tension, the corset-like transversus abdominis are able to fulfill their role of giving support.

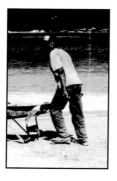 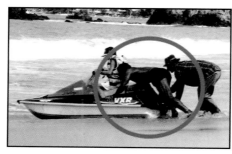 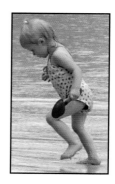

Lifting, carrying and pushing are actions that sometimes require more stabilization and core strength than ordinary activities. There are specific steps you can take to bring deeper support for the back and spine when exerting yourself in a more strenuous way.

Bracing, or bearing down through the trunk, comes naturally to people in aligned bodies. For the rest of us, the following instructions will help to locate and isolate this action.

Blow out through your mouth as if blowing out a candle, or cough a few times.

Notice the pushing-down sensation through the core of your torso. This is active engagement of the transversus abdominis muscle.

See if you can now engage this muscle when you are neither blowing out nor coughing. It has a definite bearing-down quality, like having a bowel movement or pushing out a baby.

Once you have figured out how to isolate this action in the muscle, you are able to protect yourself when lifting or pushing something heavy by maximizing this core strength with the natural strength of your arms and legs.

People with naturally aligned bodies are able to perform many tasks without excessive muscle strength. Whatever body type we have has little to do with whether or not we can perform these tasks. We can be small and thin or larger and more stout. The success of our actions depends on the strength that comes to us through a relationship of elastic muscles, aligned bones and deep core stability. Without these qualities, we are forced to overwork our bodies through great effort and muscular strain.

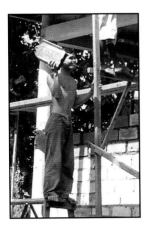 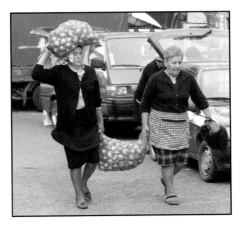 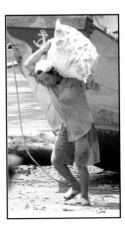

Bracing, whether done naturally or with conscious direction, stabilizes the core and prevents us from injury when lifting, carrying or pushing heavy objects.

With practice, you will be able to brace while keeping the outer belly relaxed at the same time with no interference with natural breathing.

Chapter Eleven

Implications for Health
a new prescription for the future?

What if something as simple as a chronic backward tilt of the pelvis, which mechanically establishes an inevitable compression of the spine, actually plays a role in the development of certain diseases and disorders? Recommendations for maintaining good health today are primarily focused on three primary factors: diet, stress management and exercise. What we overlook entirely is the alignment of our parts—bones, muscles and organs—and how they are designed to work together in a smooth, reliable way. Because each human body is an integrated, self-regulating process that operates through an interplay of all the body's systems, misalignment of skeletal parts, just like imprecise moving parts such as timing devices in a car engine, can throw off efficient functioning and lead to far more serious problems or breakdowns.

Until now, alignment and health have not been matched up as a topic for research. Our misunderstanding of this key component of how our bodies are designed to work, along with the mistaken belief that muscle strength is necessary to hold us up, is so widespread as to be potentially dangerous. This mistaken belief is the underlying blind spot that stands in the way of finding a key piece of a puzzle that helps explain what constitutes good health.

Good health equals normal function—no more, no less. While "normal" can sometimes refer to a culturally set standard, when it comes to health, normal means what is innate and biological—in other words, "natural." This is what we bring into the world with us and what supports our ability to thrive. If normal is interfered with, our health and well-being may suffer.

Among the essential ingredients that contribute to good health are clean air and water, nutritious food and an ability to relax and feel safe in most situations. While some unavoidable conditions—congenital disorders, certain illnesses, accidents, natural disasters—are beyond our control, many are within our realm of influence. Generally, a lack of clean air or water, a poor diet and certain conditions in our environment that leave us feeling unsafe are man-created unnatural conditions. Faulty posture is also a man-created unnatural condition.

> The growing focus on a more integrative approach to medicine arises out of an interest in a health-promoting rather than a disease-treating view of medicine. Nowhere is this more true than in the cases of millions of people who struggle with ailments that have no clear and definable cause and whose remedies continue to elude them.

Anecdotal evidence points to an important relationship that exists between skeletal alignment and health and supports principles upon which age-old traditional approaches to medicine are based:

The human body is a complex, symmetrically precise, self-regulating, interdependent process of systems, the normal state of which is homeostasis, i.e., good health.

▶ **What if OSTEOARTHRITIS were, in some cases, the result of longstanding habits of unnatural use of the body that caused repeated compression and wear and tear of joints? Could osteoarthritis be avoided in some cases and improved in others if people knew how to maintain open space and free movement in their joints?**

Osteoarthritis is characterized by degeneration and inflammation of one or more joints and is the most common reason for disability and joint replacement surgery. Symptoms can be mild to severely painful. Often termed "wear and tear" arthritis, it is commonly believed to be an inevitable consequence of aging for some people and the result of overuse of joints through certain kinds of activities for others.

Since structural misalignment and the repeated stress this places on the joints may contribute to osteoarthritis, an emphasis on realignment of bones, redistribution of the body's weight and specific movements or exercises that encourage "opening" and creation of space within the affected joint may, in some cases, bring relief. In fact, some people have found relief from symptoms by making changes in the way they sit, stand, walk and move in general.

▶   **What if a HERNIATED DISC, in many instances, is the result of chronic compression of certain segments within the cervical, thoracic or lumbar spine due to postural misalignment? It would make sense that some people might find ways to avoid developing this condition altogether or that others might learn to support the spine differently in order to find some relief from symptoms.**

The terminology describing a herniated disc can be confusing because many different terms—ruptured disc, slipped disc, pinched nerve, sciatica, bulging disc, degenerative disc disease—are sometimes used interchangeably. When diagnosing this condition, many in the medical profession tend to overlap the use of these terms, and the assessment is not always clearly discernable.

A herniated disc protrudes beyond the natural boundaries of a disc, sometimes impinging on a nerve. A ruptured disc is an extreme case, where the nucleus is squeezed beyond the wall of the disc and leaks into the spinal canal. This can be caused by traumatic injury but is far more commonly caused by habits of use that put continuous pressure on one or more discs through chronic collapse of the structure of the spine.

Not all herniated discs cause pain, and some of the ones that do, appear to repair themselves. Studies reveal that the spine lengthens in some people during the course of a night's sleep, presumably due to an increase in the water content of the disc when vertical pressure on the spine is relieved by lying down. In this way, a disc can be likened to a sponge that plumps up when it absorbs water. Squeezed dry, it flattens and becomes brittle; eventually, it crumbles and falls apart. Sometimes, discs deteriorate to the point where they can no longer re-hydrate, which can cause the facets of the vertebrae to rub against each other and generate ongoing nerve pain.

Learning how to naturally extend the spine while sitting and standing and engaging in everyday activities appears to be an obvious way to address this problem, either in terms of prevention or treatment.

▶ **What if the development of OSTEOPOROSIS were influenced, even in a small way, by one's lifelong postural habits, contributing to the creation of certain conditions that might make some people more susceptible to a process of gradual bone loss than others?**

Osteoporosis is a common condition that results in a high-level loss of bone, putting people at increased risk of fractures and general spinal deterioration. The progression of the bone loss often goes undiagnosed unless one has a bone density test or suffers a fracture. The risk of hip and spinal fractures is especially high in the older population among whom osteoporosis is particularly common. As the disease progresses, a succession of vertebral fractures, sometimes indiscernible at the time, lead to a gradual collapse of the spine and is usually accompanied by noticeable rounding of the upper back, sometimes referred to as dowager's hump. While women suffer from osteoporosis in far greater numbers than men, an estimated two million men are currently diagnosed with having this condition, and many more are at risk for developing it.

Among the generally accepted causes of osteoporosis are:

- inherited predisposition
- low calcium intake
- poor calcium absorption
- lack of weight-bearing activity
- lack of exercise
- change in reproductive hormones

It appears that no mention is ever made by anyone of the possibility that postural habits contribute, in any way, no matter how small, towards a tendency to develop osteoporosis. Curiously, however, there does seem to be an indication that at least some people who develop this condition share certain postural anomalies. Observation of people with an advanced stage of osteoporosis (a pronounced kyphotic curve) suggests that they also demonstrate a pronounced backward inclination of the pelvis, which interferes with the spine's ability to support itself. This begs the question of which came first, the backward-tilting pelvis or the collapsing spine above it? Is the progression of this disease caused by factors unrelated in any way to habitual skeletal alignment and solely by other such factors as a depletion of necessary calcium? Perhaps. While it is

131

not possible until further research is conducted to say whether postural alignment is a factor in the development of osteoporosis, the question is an important one that demands adequate examination.

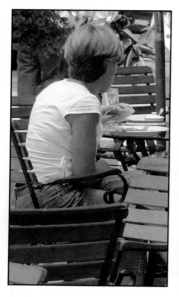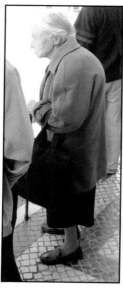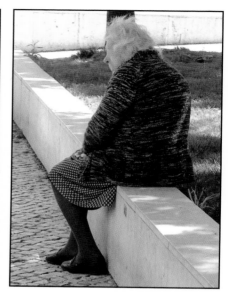

The cause of osteoporosis is unknown. While there appears to be an important link between the development of osteoporosis and what we eat—calcium intake, vitamin D, magnesium and particular types of protein all playing a part—weight-bearing exercise is also considered important. Interestingly, *how* the weight is borne by the bones, whether through bones that are aligned or bones that are not, has not been considered much of a factor. Over the course of decades, it is conceivable that this could, in fact, play an important role.

Research that examines the postural habits of people who develop osteoporosis could lead towards new understanding of how various causes might overlap and interplay with one another. While some studies have been conducted that compare the incidence of osteoporosis among different cultures, the emphasis has primarily been on diet and lifestyle, not longstanding structural habits of support. Studies that track the bone density and postural habits of people diagnosed with osteopenia (early stage bone loss) could potentially reveal whether adopting new habits of posture plays an important preventive role.

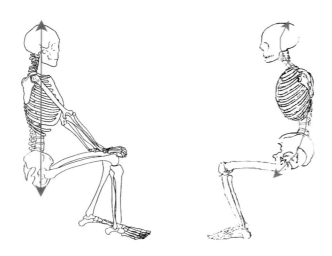

> **What if skeletal alignment plays a role, either large or small, in other musculoskeletal disorders such as KYPHOSIS, LORDOSIS or various back conditions such as SPONDYLOSIS and other generalized types of back pain?**

Kyphosis is the name given to excessive rounding of the thoracic spine, or upper back. Lordosis, which is sometimes referred to as swayback, is excessive arching of the lumbar spine. Spondylosis is osteoarthritis of the spine and its facet joints. All of these conditions can cause varying degrees of pain and discomfort as well as accelerated aging. In a study of the literature pertaining to these conditions, they appear to have no known cause. This can be frustrating not only for people in pain but also for their doctors, who are often at a loss to know how to treat them other than through medication or surgery.

Some people who have "tried everything," have found ways to release some of their pain themselves by directing their attention to how they are inhabiting their body and learning ways to release tension and pain from the inside out. For those who find this approach works well for them, it can come as a surprise to discover that hardly any research is being done that examines the relationship between the skeleton's alignment and back pain.

While the relationship between skeletal alignment and disorders affecting the musculoskeletal system may seem logical, other conditions—particularly those having to do with dysfunction of the nervous, cardiovascular and respiratory systems—may seem more improbable. However, closer examination reveals that there are several ways in which one's alignment could potentially affect the smooth functioning of other systems of the body.

▶ What if skeletal alignment plays a role in certain RESPIRATORY DISORDERS, influenced by whether or not diaphragmatic muscle fibers are in a natural configuration or if they are askew. This might affect their ability to contract and relax in a natural, efficient way. Taking into account the growing body of evidence that CHRONIC HYPERVENTILATION SYNDROME plays a role in stress-related disorders such as ANXIETY and PANIC ATTACKS, while also frequently mimicking symptoms of chest pain and heart attack, research into this area is vital.

Stress kills. It does this by triggering sympathetic nervous system dominance and interfering with the immune system's ability to ward off infections and diseases. It is still unclear from a purely scientific perspective what role, if any, skeletal alignment might play in contributing to chronic stress to the nervous system. This sort of involvement, if it were shown to have an effect, would be by way of distortion of the diaphragm and compression of the spinal cord as seen in typical skeletal collapse and slouching, or conversely through "lifting and holding" oneself upward.

Because researchers limit their observations to third person subjects and do not become the subjects of their own experiments, certain details that can only be discovered through direct experience may never rise to the surface as points worthy of examination. Nevertheless, just about anyone will experience this tension along the spine simply by tucking under the tailbone, sucking in the belly, lifting up the chest and raising up the chin. This engages the "fight or flight" response—stopped breathing and a heightened state of tension and alert.

The resulting tension that is felt along the spine may well serve as a "button" that, for some people, is constantly being pressed to turn the sympathetic nervous system "on." This chronic, low-level state of alarm appears to be the condition many people live in much of the time. Some of the alarm may well be due to something as simple as the position of their bones.

People who learn how to shift their way of being in their bodies from ram-rod straight and held up find it comes as a great relief to let their bones support them.

They can finally relax and stop working so hard. One can feel the parasympathetic nervous system flood the body with the relaxation response as the belly relaxes, the chest settles down and lungs appear to "breathe for themselves."

Beyond the subjective experience of the link between skeletal alignment and the nervous system, there has been essentially no scientific research whatsoever that examines any possible relationship.

▶ **What if skeletal alignment plays a role in the overall health of the CARDIOVASCULAR SYSTEM, dictating to some extent whether veins and arteries are fully open—like tiny garden hoses—or that might at times be crimped by chronic slouching or narrowed by hyperextended, uplifted posture?**

Patients with high-blood pressure or other cardiovascular conditions are told to watch their intake of cholesterol and fats, to exercise regularly and to sometimes take medication to control their blood pressure. Rarely, if ever, is a patient's structural alignment considered in terms of how it might affect how efficiently blood moves through the arteries and veins, delivering life-giving oxygen and nutrients to cells and transporting wastes and toxins away from the cells, to be released from the body. While there is no evidence that this is so, might there be a possibility that plaque would be more likely to accumulate—the way silt does in a pipe—in those parts of an artery that are chronically narrowed by collapsed posture?

What if something as mechanically simple as the core structural components of the body play a part—in addition to other key factors such as heredity, diet, stress level and lifestyle—in establishing conditions of overall health for the organism? What if structural alignment fulfills the role of a finely tuned instrument in an orchestra of many instruments, performing in an interplay of systems to contribute to a smooth-playing whole?

Chapter Twelve

Beyond the Physical
finding peace inside a body

Learning the mechanical details of the human body's design and applying them to our own selves can open other possibilities far beyond just the physical elements involved. Natural alignment is also a place, a quality of being into which one relaxes. It can be experienced physically, mentally, emotionally and spiritually and comes with a sense of recognition, a coming home to what is inborn and unchanging. It taps into the essence of who and what we always are.

For us to recognize this place, we must turn our attention inward, underneath our skin, and invite a process of gradual unfolding through directed awareness. Although we may find support and encouragement from others who are doing or have done the same, no one else can do this for us, on us or to us. Going within is strictly a solo act. In the end, it is up to each one of us, if we choose, to discover what it means to be human in a moment-by-moment way.

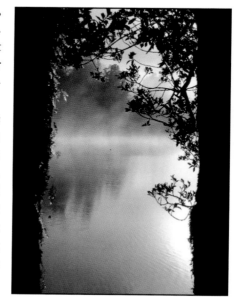

This is not an easy thing to do because being aware of our present experience means that we will sometimes encounter tension and pain, both physical and nonphysical. Almost everyone's tendency is to want to avoid whatever makes us uncomfortable. We want joy, not sadness; security, not fear; pleasure, not pain. Most of us will do just about anything in the pursuit of the first and avoidance of the second.

We read a book, watch TV, go to a movie, work overtime, call a friend, take a vacation, open a beer, have a snack, go to the mall, surf the net, take a nap, watch more TV, have another snack…None of these activities is wrong or bad. They are common, normal everyday activities that anyone should feel free to enjoy. The problem arises when we relentlessly stack one on top of another and yet another, until we have limited our ability to tune in with awareness to what it might mean to be a human "being," rather than a human "doing." We are often unaware that some of our strategies for avoiding tension and pain are at the root of what might be causing it in the first place.

Avoiding pain only leads to more pain, in most cases, whether mental, emotional or physical. Pain is a signal, a call to attention from which we typically deny or run away. We hope it will go away, and so we busy ourselves to keep our minds engaged elsewhere. Sometimes, we can hide out from pain indefinitely, but usually, it is only a matter of time before it returns. One effective way to address this situation is to develop greater awareness through a practice of mindfulness. Mindfulness is simply being aware of one's present experience in an ongoing process of investigation and discovery. One observes experiences as they occur and as one is participating in them, without judgment.

Simply deciding that we are going to be mindful is not enough, however, as anyone who tries to put this into practice soon learns. Mindfulness can only be contacted in each moment, and in the beginning, more often than not, it is lost in the next.

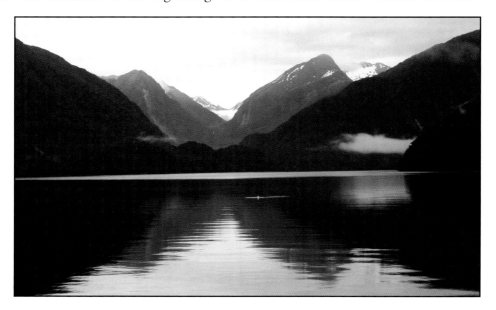

Mindfulness meditation is a specific practice designed, in part, to help train the mind to be more aware. Awareness can have an elusive quality to it, perhaps because of years spent not focusing the mind in this way. Whenever we make an effort to pay attention to the rising and falling of the breath or the sensations of the body, we may realize at some point that our mind has wandered away again. Our attempt at paying attention was short lived. We might try again, still without success, and then decide our minds are too active for this and give up.

If we do not give up, but instead keep returning to the breath again and again, it won't be long before we start to develop fortitude, a quality we will need for this practice. Mindfulness meditation has proven to be so effective in reducing stress and improving health that this technique has now been successfully incorporated into hundreds of hospital programs around the United States. On the physical level, it appears to work by turning down the volume on the sympathetic aspect of the nervous system while allowing the parasympathetic aspect (relaxation response) to play a more balanced role.

> **Focusing your awareness on any of the details of natural alignment—the position of the three wheels, extension through the spine, a belly that is relaxed—can serve as an easily accessible, concrete tool for anchoring your awareness to the present moment.**

Good News/Bad News

When dealing with self-directed change and how one inhabits the body, there is good news and bad news. The bad news is that you must be, forever and always, mindful. The good news is that you must be, forever and always, mindful! Paying close attention to how you are sitting, standing, bending, walking, breathing, tensing, relaxing—noticing, noticing, noticing—is one of the most difficult and challenging undertakings you will ever encounter. At the same time, this practice brings with it benefits that far outweigh any of the difficulties initially encountered. Many people report positive changes that include improved health and greater peace of mind.

While the formalized practice of mindfulness meditation is not a requirement for re-learning how to be naturally aligned, mindfulness as a quality of your daily life is essential. In fact, learning to align your bones is, simply put, an awareness practice. The sad or happy truth, depending on how you look at it, is that there simply is no short cut for paying attention in the moment. In any given moment, your attention is either here and now, or it is not. You are either aware of how you are sitting (or standing, walking, breathing, etc.), or you are not.

> In this never-ending process of remembering and then forgetting to be present, it is our willingness to begin—again and again and again—and simply noticing without judgment that rests at the very heart of this practice.

Judging ourselves for forgetting only creates more tension. Letting go of our judgments is translated into letting go of the tensions, both physical and nonphysical, that hold us captive and prevent us from knowing peace. The more quiet and present we become, the more we notice that each thought, each emotion and action creates tension.

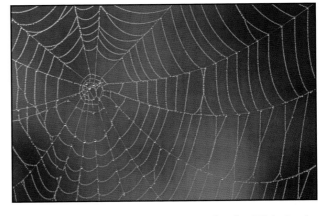

It can be easy to imagine that the way to arrive at some realm of enlightenment is by transcending a body that is commonly viewed as mundane, earthbound, clumsy, even at times repulsive and, on top of all that, causes us pain. Yet, any legitimate road to a loftier, more spiritual existence is one that leads inward, right back into the body, not beyond it.

Initially at least, it is not that I have a body, but that I am a body. This is the reality of everyone's existence in time and space. Where I run into trouble is when I identify this body as being uniquely 'my own' as a stand-alone, disconnected entity that defines me as being separate. Because everyone is a body, almost everyone has an opportunity to consciously inhabit that body in all the ordinary messiness of everyday life. In doing so, we might discover that we are not so separate after all.

This body is where life is lived. How else would we ever know we are sad if we did not feel sad? Or joyful? Or tired? Any time we are angry, we know without any doubt, that anger is, first and foremost, a physical experience. While it may be a thought that triggers a certain emotion, the emotion itself is a felt one, thus it is called a feeling. When we run away from our feelings, when we are too busy and preoccupied to know what they even are, we lose out on living our lives fully, whether our moments come with joy, sorrow, pain, pleasure or equanimity. Our transformation—from pain to no pain, (or at least, less pain) and from turmoil to peace—comes through the body, not away from it. Something as seemingly ordinary as aligning one's bones or sensing the rising and falling of the breath becomes an essential tool for anchoring our awareness in this moment, no matter what might be going on around us. The more we explore and discover what natural alignment actually means, the more we connect with and wake up to our thoughts and feelings, our physical sensations and all the possibilities of experience that reside within.

In these quiet moments of awareness when we notice what is actually happening in and around and through us, it is not the body that is transcended but the separation of body, mind and spirit. "The power of now" is a concept that has stirred great interest recently through a popular book by that title (See Endnotes). Consciously inhabiting the body, of which awareness of aligned skeletal support is one essential part, is the power of now.

Body as Metaphor

Words inspire the imagination and draw pictures in the mind. The words "he is full of himself" most likely will conjure up an image of someone with a puffed-up chest and whose energetic presence is directed into the front of the body (head and rib cage wheels rolled backward). This is a different image than the one seen by the mind's eye when hearing someone described as being spineless, having no backbone or weak-kneed (rib cage wheel forward and pelvic wheel back). Someone can be a pain in the neck because she keeps a stiff upper lip, has feet of clay, is an anal-retentive tight ass (pelvic wheel rolled backward), and turns a deaf ear. Again, this is not the same as having your head in the clouds and therefore, not having a leg to stand on. These are not just random expressions that landed in our language but windows into the body that, at times, offer a glimpse into psychological and emotional aspects of a person's being.

Chances are you look quite different when you are feeling depressed and "low" than you do when you are feeling excited and "up." Then again, there is the middle way of equanimity—neither up nor down but centered—where the bones are aligned and the energy is calm. The fundamental energy that is the ground of our being and exists as a never-ending stream of consciousness at any given moment is either flowing freely or is bogged down someplace. Our skeletal alignment plays a vital role in setting up conditions that facilitate our ability to participate in this flow.

Accomplished actors draw upon subtle details of skeletal alignment in creating the characters their bodies temporarily inhabit. Someone who is stuck up and looks down her nose at people is arrogant and has a condescending attitude. She also has a chin that is lifted upward, this being a requirement for being able to look down her nose in the first place. Physically, this creates compression in the cervical part of her spine and tension in muscles of the neck that interrupt the natural, easy flow of energy, causing blockage and constriction instead.

Of course, we must be careful not to make sweeping generalizations that oversimplify a complex issue that may be beyond our understanding. So many other factors are involved in contributing to the totality of our physical and emotional being. Obviously, many people who have a chronically lifted chin might not have a condescending attitude. Every one of them, however, does have compression in the cervical spine that blocks the flow of vital energy.

Whatever kinds of psychic tensions result from this may or may not contribute to a particular attitude of mind or body. Curiously, attitude, while meaning "having a particular perspective on something," also means "taking a certain physical posture, especially while interacting with others." Over and over again, we find cues in our language that point to the fact that the connections between mind and body have been understood by many who came before us. It may be only in recent history that we have become disconnected enough from our center to lose sight of this fact.

Sometimes, our bodies reflect our moods or the tendencies of our varied personalities. When the skeleton is pushed forward of the central axis, it can be said that one has the appearance of living in the future, striving toward goals and checking off a "to-do" list. When our bodies reflect this stature, we might have expectations and be preoccupied with planning and fantasizing. A lifted chest can give the impression we are at least putting up a good front of confidence. If the spine and chest are collapsed, it could

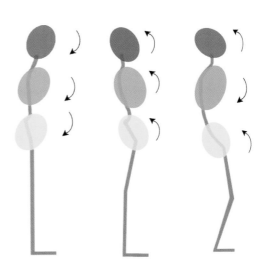

be said we are dwelling in the past, in the land of regrets. "If only" might be words that begin sentences that are born out of a mind that is ruled by memories.

Often, when we are caught hanging onto past hurts and such, our body might take on a punched-in-the-stomach appearance. For some people, this has become a chronic condition. Off-center skeletons are not aligned, at least physically, with the present. Awareness of the present seems to be more typically reflected in a body that lives easily and fluidly in line with the central axis—the middle way—in a physical manifestation of simple acceptance of what is.

Somewhere between fighting against gravity and being defeated by it, between holding one's head up too high and collapsing under the weight of a head full of worries is a middle way of being. This middle path comes from living in the present with an acceptance that moves us from the loss and hurt of the past to the seductive anticipation of a brighter future. Acceptance heals our sorrows, mends our fences and reveals the silver linings. Acceptance gives birth to humility, a quality of grace that is sometimes revealed in the naturally aligned body with a chest that is soft and vulnerable, not tight and guarded (rib cage wheel rolling forward, not back).

It is common to think that lifting and "opening" the chest forward is the same as consciously opening the heart. However, when the chest is opened outward in the front, this heart we are trying to open is physically constricted by tension in the back. This compassionate heart is a three-dimensional, spiraling vortex of chakra energy that spins around that same central axis, requiring centered alignment for it as well as all chakras to be open. The energetic spine in the yogic tradition—*sushumna nadi*—corresponds to the physical spine. For one to be fully open, the other must be as well.

Perhaps a truly open heart is one that opens out equally in all directions, in a metaphorical inclusiveness that matches what the heart is all about. Lifting up the chest can also be experienced as lifting a shield up to protect ourselves from being hurt, the pain of which every one of us knows only too well. It takes centered awareness to put down the shield. The compassion we develop for others is born out of acknowledgement of our own pain. When we close off the physical heart, when it is pinched and tight, it may be difficult for us to bring compassion forward, whether for ourselves or for others. Putting down the physical/emotional shield means we are willing to be vulnerable, to risk being hurt, to love unconditionally and forgive ourselves and each other for all things. This is the humility of an open heart, manifested in a human body.

The Psycho-Spiritual Center of Gravity

Consciously turning our attention inward and reestablishing our alignment along the central axis can bring about remarkable changes in our emotional and psychological state. It is not necessary for us to understand the cause of the problem so much as the solution to it. Herein lies the wisdom of "letting go." Developing an ability to be mindful of each moment, of the body and of the breath, without judgment, will help guide us back to home base. Uncomfortable situations that once frightened us may be more easily resolved from this center.

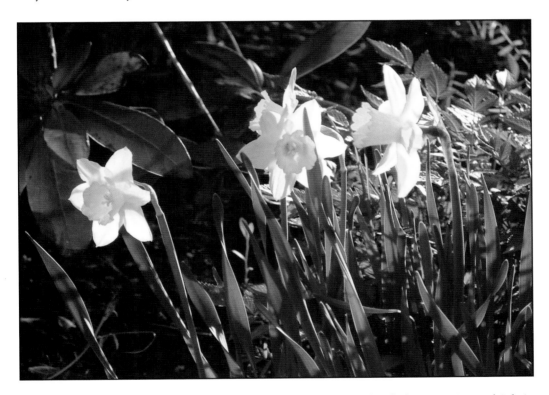

Although "real" in the world of Newtonian physics, this balance point, which is located along the central axis, cannot be seen or touched. It is not a particle or even a molecule, and while it is mysteriously invisible, it can still be calculated and measured. This center of gravity is also an experience, one that can only be understood directly through the experience of the body. It is a taproot to our deepest sense of being, the point where body, mind, and spirit converge.

Not only is this home base located along the central axis or line of gravity, its very center rests precisely at a point in the center of the belly, below the navel and halfway between the front and the back of the abdomen. This is the balance point for the body, our virtual center of gravity. The point through which the sum of gravitational forces on a body can be considered to act is not just a physical reality called the center of gravity.

In Japan, this is called Hara; in China, it is the Tan Tien. None of the European languages appear to have a word that captures the ineffable, energetic quality of this physical center. Gut feeling, while falling short, is the closest expression found in English that describes an intuitive sort of knowing that is beyond rational thought. Once again, words we sometimes use without understanding their origins tell the story of what some of our ancestors might have known that we have long since forgotten.

"Gut feelings" can be difficult to experience when they are locked inside "killer abs." We live in a culture that reveres abdominal muscles. Even mannequins modeling bathing suits in store windows proudly display flat, rippling abs. Many health-related magazines will have at least one article per issue on how to flatten your belly in ten days or less. Unfortunately, many of the exercises designed to do this only entrench tension patterns that repeatedly compress the spine and tighten the diaphragm, thus restricting natural, relaxed breathing. As a culture, we are binding ourselves up with more and more tension when our greatest freedom lies in the boundless peace available to us when those tensions are released.

> " 'Chest out—belly in'...a nation capable of taking this injunction as a general rule is in great danger," said a Japanese to me in 1938. It was during my first visit to Japan. I did not understand this sentence then. Today I know it is true, and why.'
> —Karlfried Graf Durkheim, *Hara: The Vital Center of Man*, 1956

Our greatest strength and power lie in the belly, not in a belly that is tight and closed off to the flow of energy but one that is relaxed and open to the life force moving through it. The billions of cells in our body are fed by a breath that is born in a soft and receptive belly. We think the breath comes into us from outside, but that is only the physical aspect of drawing in oxygen. The breath, that profound mystery of physical existence that bridges life and death, is born deep within us and teaches us how to live and how to die as we watch it rise up from the depths, then fall away, only to be born and to die again and again. By returning our awareness to this "abdominal brain," we may connect with an earth wisdom that is our birthright, which feeds the heights of our consciousness the same way deep roots feed a tall tree.

As humans, we are perfectly positioned between heaven and earth. Transcending our earthly weight depends on our capacity to let go and surrender to the earth, taking delight in our connection and letting all tensions drop away. In answer to this yielding, a response of gentle rising through the central axis can be experienced, both mechanically and energetically, much as in Newton's Third Law, which postulates that for every action there is an opposite and equal reaction. We realize that heaven is not some far-off future place but is a condition we can experience right here, right now. We gain admission to heaven when we do not deny or betray the earth. A soft "Buddha belly" promotes this connection, and naturally aligned bones let us know we are always safe and supported, even when we relax. Without the security of aligned bones, we will collapse when we relax.

To counter this tendency toward collapse, the present culture of health and fitness may have gone too far in thinking that in terms of belly muscles, flatter is stronger, stronger is better and better is more. "More" takes us out of balance, away from a state of equilibrium where all the interconnected parts of the whole (holons) function in an optimal arrangement of working parts. Too much over here has to mean not enough over there, a maxim that applies as equally to the balanced action of bones and muscles as it does to a world that has great disparity between "haves" and "have nots."

The remarkable thing about the underlying mystery that governs this universe is that it can never be measured or observed in order to be understood; it must be experienced. By shifting our perspective from that of disconnected observer to that of consciously living, breathing participants, an interconnected, unbroken wholeness reveals itself as the universal intelligence that governs everything. Beyond thought, beyond reason, we simply understand.

As far-flung from the function of the abdominal muscles as this discussion may seem, it lies at the absolute heart of why it behooves us to relax our bellies and align our bones. By doing so, we once again become participants and not just observers. We release the tensions that have prevented us from tapping into the flow of life, consciously opening channels through which the pulse of life merges with itself. Any self-studying scientist can simply put this to the test by sucking in and holding in the belly, while noticing the feeling, then releasing it slowly, and noticing again.

Coming Home to Peace

Is it possible that the message of all the great spiritual teachers is simply to relax in a profoundly deep and caring way? To open ourselves to the flow of life by letting go of all tensions of the mind and body that stand in our way? Could the instruction "Except ye be as little children, ye shall in no way enter the Kingdom of Heaven" be a call to trust and yield, to live in the moment with full awareness of the glorious present? What might this look like in a body?

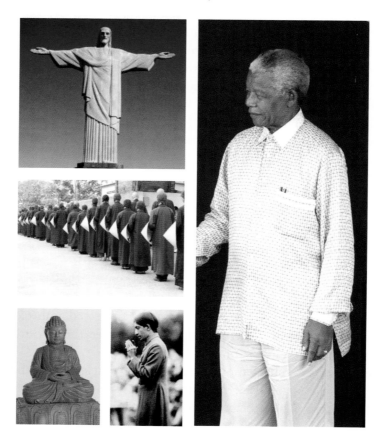

Profoundly peaceful people seem to embody certain qualities. Most paintings and statues of Jesus depict him as having a body that aligns itself along the central axis. These images are man-made, of course, but the artists creating them might have found it hard to imagine Jesus walking around with a slouching, collapsed posture or, conversely, with his chest lifted upward and pushed out in front. It's equally hard to imagine Jesus sporting over-developed muscles underneath his robes.

The same holds true for the Buddha, Jiddu Krishnamurti, Nelson Mandela and others who, like Jesus, epitomize humility, forgiveness and peace. All reflect a naturally aligned and relaxed body. Whether sitting or standing, Jesus, the Buddha and others (as we imagine them) are the picture of tranquility and acceptance. Translated into physical details, this would mean an aligned skeleton and relaxed belly, something that is not only available to those who have a publicly-recognized spiritual presence but to anyone and everyone of us by virtue of the fact that we are human beings with human bodies.

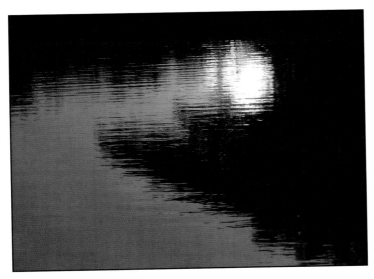

"I feel it in my bones" are words that tell of an ancient intuition pointing to the connection between a physical body and a quantum mind and leads all the way inside to the marrow of the universe. Just as there is release from the tensions of the body/mind when thoughts and emotions align with an acceptance of "what is," there is also release from the tensions of the body/mind when the bones align with the reality of our biomechanical design.

When we are keenly aware of our own internal life, our consciousness becomes more permeable, allowing new possibilities to seep in. We discover that we are all a part of the same whole, the same light force, the same energy. The multidimensional aspects of the human being are all aligned with this whole. By embodying presence, we discover that we are not so much traveling a path as we are the path.

PART II

A Self-Guided Tour

There is deep wisdom within our very flesh,

if we can only come to our senses and feel it.

Elizabeth Behnke

PUTTING ALIGNMENT INTO PRACTICE

In order to learn how to sit, stand, bend and otherwise inhabit the body in a naturally relaxed way, we must first understand how key parts of the body relate to each other. The following Explorations are designed to do just that. It is important to start at the beginning and work through each one sequentially, as they build one upon the other. Once these are understood, we can apply them to everyday activities such as sitting, standing, and bending.

Patience and an open mind are necessary ingredients for this to take hold. Some of the instructions may be quite opposite from what you believe to be true. Cultural conditioning is pervasive, and consequently certain movement patterns are deeply set in the mind as well as the body. Some people say the changes feel weird compared to what has always felt familiar. It is helpful to remember that just because a way of inhabiting your body is normal for you, it is not necessarily natural. Taking these instructions into your own body might cause you to feel like you are slouching a bit, especially if you like almost everyone else have been taught to sit and stand up straight by tucking your tailbone and lifting your chest. It helps to keep in mind that this is a stage you might have to pass through that normally does not last very long.

At no time should you feel any pain when making these adjustments. Sometimes, a pulling sensation may occur, as chronically tight muscles are being asked to lengthen after being on vacation for decades. It is important to distinguish between a pinch and a pull. A pinch may be your body telling you to back off. If this happens, you may want to reread the instructions and try again. If a pinching pain continues, stop. Refer to the Appendix for help.

IMPORTANT POINTS TO REMEMBER

- Reestablishing alignment along the central axis is not a quick fix. It took many years for familiar habits of use to become embedded in your muscle fibers and your psyche. It will take time and consistent practice to consciously override these default settings. The rewards are well worth it.

- Patience and a commitment to be mindful are essential. Without this, change will be impossible. In this case, practice does not make perfect so much as practice makes for more practice. Do not think of this as a goal so much as taking aim in a more natural direction.

- These instructions may seem simplistic at first or too different from what is already familiar to you. The following instructions may represent a departure from what you believe to be true.

- These instructions may be difficult for some people to learn from a book. Some habits are beyond the reach of the conscious mind. Keep trying. If this does not work for you, refer to the Appendix to find a Balance teacher who can help show you how to override longstanding practices.

- Make use of any therapies and modalities that support you in becoming more aligned and relaxed. If possible, avoid those forms of exercise and activities (at least for now) that reinforce unhelpful habits. At some point down the road, you may be able to participate in these activities in a way that is natural and safe.

- Doing this becomes easier with time. DON'T GIVE UP! The payoff is relief from pain, greater ease and comfort, improved health and vitality, more graceful aging and greater awareness in each moment.

RINGING THE BELLS OF ALIGNMENT

The image of bells ringing in a tower makes it easy to sense the different ways in which the pelvis, rib cage and head are able to move. This is a simplified version of the Three Wheels, that is a good place to start when first applying these concepts to our own bodies. The wheels approach is a refinement of this action that is more useful for understanding how these bony parts affect the length of the spine. More about this later.

For now, we'll begin to imagine these parts—the pelvis, rib cage and head—as bells. Of course, if these were real bells, all the clappers on the two outside figures would hang straight down. For our purposes here, they have been left suspended in order to better demonstrate the angle of distortion of the spine's trajectory.

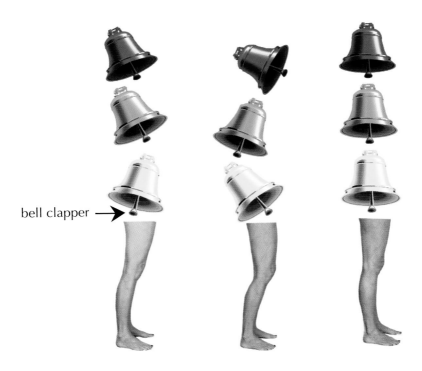

bell clapper ⟶

EXPLORATION #1 LOCATING THE PELVIC LANDMARKS

Pubic Bone
or Pubis Symphisis

Sit bones
or ischial tuberosities,
the balance points on
which the pelvis rests

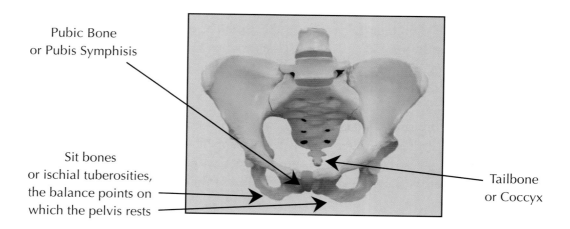

Tailbone
or Coccyx

- Begin by sitting on a chair with a level seat (or forward on the edge of a chair) with both feet flat on the floor. Place one or both hands underneath you, and let your weight come down onto your fingers. Roll around on your fingers until you feel the bony knobs, or ischial tuberosities. (Hint: if you can't find them, move your hands forward and closer to the midline). These are commonly called the "sit bones."

- The second landmark is the pubis symphysis, or pubic bone. Located at the front of the pelvis, this is where two bones of the pelvis meet, separated by cartilage.

- The third landmark is the coccyx, or tailbone. This appears to be a residual tail, left over from long-ago ancestors.

EXPLORATION #2 RINGING THE PELVIC BELL

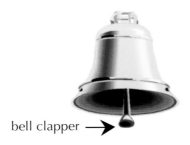

bell clapper ➔

- Stand with your heels six inches apart and your toes eight inches apart. Move your thighs forward, in front of you, then back behind you. Repeat this movement, and notice how this causes the pelvis to move like a bell swinging in a church tower.

- Notice that when the pubic bone moves forward and up, the sit bones follow, moving closer to each other at the same time. When the pubic bone moves down and behind you, the sit bones move back and apart. Caution: Do not let the sit bones rise up behind you since this will cause unnecessary tension in the lower back and hips. Let them simply slide out straight behind you. Notice how the tailbone moves along with the sit bones and pubis.

- Repeat this movement slowly, paying close attention to any sensations you observe. These may include tightening and releasing of muscles in the front and back of the thighs, the hips joints, the buttocks and the belly. Notice the sensations in the floor of the pelvis—how it tightens and narrows when the pubic bone rises up in front, then opens and relaxes as the pubic bone moves down again.

- Find the neutral resting place where the floor of the pelvis is as relaxed as possible where you have a sense of the "bell clapper" hanging straight down.

EXPLORATION #3 STANDING EXPLORATION

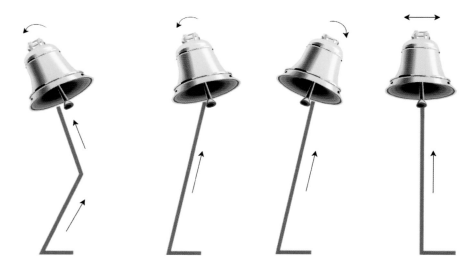

- Stand in front of a full-length mirror. Turn to the side and observe the alignment of your legs. Are they straight and perpendicular? Or are they angled in one direction or another?

- As you slowly lean to move your thighs out in front of you and then to the back, notice how the positions of your legs change. Remember that you need long, straight columns of support underneath you when you stand. Do this again and notice how the position of the pelvis changes to match the bells in the above drawings. Do this one more time and notice how the angle of your ankles changes.

- As you continue to move your legs and swing the pelvic bell, notice how the weight shifts onto your heels and your legs become long and straight. This is a neutral pelvis. If you feel like you are going to tip backwards on your heels, don't go quite so far. This is common when leg muscles have not been working adequately to hold you up all these years. This unstable feeling will change when you practice this regularly.

- Relax your belly. CAUTION: Do not let the sit bones rise up behind you since this will cause tension in the lower back and hips.

EXPLORATION #7 HOME BASE FOR THE RIB CAGE

- Establish your SOLID SEAT (Exploration #4) on the sit bones. Make sure the pelvis remains stable and unmoving at all times. This will set your foundation and allow you to release the rib cage without collapse.

- Slowly swing the rib cage 'bell' back and forth several or more times (again, the pelvis does not move!). Pay close attention to the shifting length in the line along the front and then the back of your body. As the bottom of the bell swings behind you, the line in the front shortens and your back rounds; as the bottom of the bell swings to the front, the back arches and the chest pushes out. CAUTION: Only go as far as this is comfortable.

- Can you sense how this movement is reflected in your spine? Can you feel your spine compress on whichever side the line is shortening? Can you find a middle place, where the line is the same length in the front and the back? Keep relaxing the belly. Are you able to tell that the spine is optimally extended when both lines are the same length?

- You may have to remind the belly to relax many times over. Chronic tension in abdominal muscles is a big part of what keeps the rib cage and pelvis 'glued' together. A relaxed belly allows the pelvis and rib cage to move independently of each other.

- You may sense a corset-like action in muscles all around the waist as you do this. This tension will be different from the sucking in the belly kind of tension you may be used to. This bracing action, when done correctly, anchors the pubic bone and sit bones, as the transversus abdominis muscle engages instead of the rectus abdominis muscles. Understanding how this works may take some practice. Be patient with yourself.

EXPLORATION #8 FINDING LENGTH THRU THE SPINE

Learning to release the rib cage from a held up, backward rolling position takes practice. Besides the fact that muscle patterns are often deeply entrenched in our bodies, it can be hard to accept, after all we have been taught about "good" posture, that the way to lengthen the spine is to let the chest sink down in front.

One way to experience optimal length through the spine is to first establish your SOLID SEAT (Exploration #4) on the sit bones with an unmoving pelvis planted on a chair. Place your fingers at the base of the breastbone (sternum), and guide the breastbone towards your back and up behind you (forward-rolling rib cage wheel). Can you feel your spine lengthen through the center of your torso as your upper back rises? Your shoulders will lift up and come forward. Don't worry about this—we will learn what to do with the shoulders in the next exploration. The focus of this particular exercise is simply to experience the full length of the spine up through the center of your core.

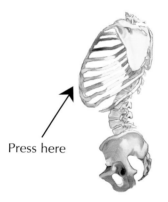

Press here

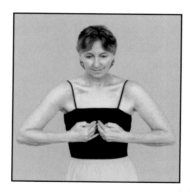

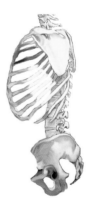

Once the spine is fully lengthened, imagine that you are placing your upper back onto a high shelf immediately behind you. Notice how this creates optimal length from your hips to your arm pits, with the center of the arm pits lifting straight up. Maintain this length through your spine as you release your shoulders down, one at a time, onto the top of the rib cage.

EXPLORATION #9 SHOULDER ROLLS

• Establish your SOLID SEAT (Exploration #4).

• Drop your chest as your upper back rises up behind you.

• Lift your right shoulder up, then roll it back and down, letting it come to rest right on top of the rib cage.

• Repeat on the left side. Make sure that you keep your rib cage settled down in front at all times. Always roll only one shoulder at a time in order to avoid triggering deep habitual patterns that undo the natural suspension of the rib cage.

• It helps to know that you can turn your palm up and down without moving the upper arm or shoulder as the action takes place below the elbow. This can feel strange at first if you are in the habit of moving your hand all the way from your shoulder. Knowing this can help you learn to release chronic shoulder strain and tension.

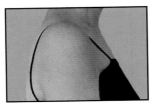 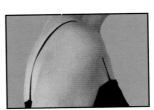

Shoulder dropped forward   Aligned shoulder resting
off of rib cage   on top of rib cage

EXPLORATION #10 A GOOD HEAD ON THOSE SHOULDERS

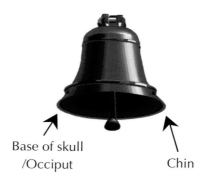

Base of skull
/Occiput   Chin

The image of a bell works well for initially exploring the basic up/down ("yes") movement of the atlanto-occipital joint, where the head rests on top of the spine. When the head 'bell' swings forward, the chin comes up; when the bell swings back, the chin drops down toward the throat and the base of the skull rises up behind.

Once again, it is essential that the bones below be in place.

Establish your SOLID SEAT (Exploration #4), relax the belly, let the chest drop in front as the mid-back rises up and then, one at a time, roll your shoulders.

Begin by slowly lifting the chin. Only the head moves. Avoid any movement of the chest or torso. Can you sense the shortening and arching of the cervical (neck) part of the spine as the chin lifts? Take this far enough so that you actually feel how the weight of the head bears down on the antlanto-occipital joint. CAUTION: Do not do this if it causes any pain.

Very slowly, drop the chin down toward your throat, paying close attention to the sensations of the spine as it lengthens and rises up through the neck.

Let your awareness rest with the small muscles that attach at the topmost vertebrae and the base of the skull (occiput). Notice the sensations of these muscles shortening as the chin rises and the sensations of them lengthening as the chin drops down.

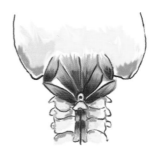

Another way to experience this movement of your head is to imagine the top of the head being partially filled with sand, like a large egg timer lying on its side. When you lift the chin, the sand pours into the back of the head.

Slowly drop your chin all the way to the chest, and feel the sand pour into the front of the skull. You'll be looking at your chest.

Let the up and down movements become smaller as you pay attention to the sensation in the neck as the sand begins to tip toward the back of the head. Feel how the weight jams down onto the atlanto-occipital joint and the neck muscles have to work to hold up all this weight. Explore the middle place, where the sand appears to be equally balanced between front and back and the muscles of the neck are optimally relaxed. Lift the head back up starting from the base of the neck. Relaxing the belly will help relax the neck.

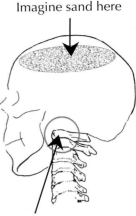

Imagine sand here

Atlano-occipital joint

GOOSE NECK

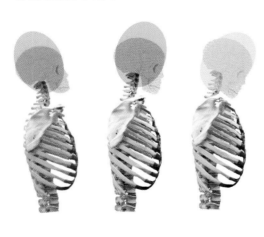

Extend your chin way out in front of you, then drop it down towards your chest. Slowly, begin to roll the chin up the front of your throat. Keep your chest down. The moment you feel tension arising anywhere, pause. Relax the belly, then continue to roll the chin upward until you feel more tension arising. Relax the belly again, and continue to roll the chin up this way. This is a helpful exercise for aligning and releasing the neck as long as you succeed in relaxing.

OPEN YOUR EYES

If you feel that your eyes are aimed at the floor in front of you, look up with your eyes rather than lifting your chin. Expect this to feel strange at first, as you will be using your eye muscles differently. Lifting the chin causes the eyelids to close slightly. Dropping your chin slightly means you will be looking out at the world with your eyes wide open!

EXPLORATION #11 STANDING SOLIDLY ON TWO FEET

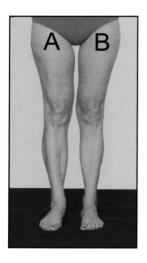

Side A in the photo shows a foot that does not provide adequate support for the leg or the entire body above it. The ankle is dropping inward off the ankle platform, the arch is collapsed, the weight is thrown onto the inside of the heel, the toes are weak and ineffective, both the knee and hip are unsupported. This leg has an unengaged appearance that reflects a general lack of vitality.

Side B shows aligned foot bones, a healthy arch, a stabilized ankle and knee, dynamic toes and active, healthy tonus of the muscles throughout the leg.

The difference between these two legs is striking, with each foot setting the stage (literally) for what is possible for the leg and body above it.

Aligning Feet and Legs While Wearing Shoes

Foot scoops (see the next section) are an exercise for the feet that help train the muscles to support the leg and ankle in a naturally aligned way by arranging the bones of the feet to their proper position. Foot scoops are done in bare feet and temporarily rearrange the bones of the feet to their natural place.

To align the legs while wearing shoes, stand with heels six inches apart and toes eight inches apart. Roll both knees and thighs outward from the center. Do this by keeping both knees straight (but not locked) and turning your knees away from each other. If you think of your legs as pillars on which you stand, this action rotates each pillar outward. Like foot scoops, this action also engages the muscles that lift the arches and keep the legs active and working. CAUTION: Do not let this action cause the tailbone to tuck under. Orthotic arches can be helpful in some cases. (See Appendix).

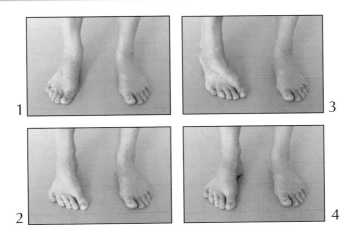

FOOT SCOOPS

You may want to do this in front of a mirror in order to see the change in your legs and feet.

Figure 1: Stand with heels six inches apart and toes eight inches apart.

Figure 2: Lift the heel of the right foot slightly, and turn the toes toward the left.

Figure 3: Holding onto the floor with the toes and the ball of the foot, roll the right knee and thigh away from the center (to the right), bringing the heel in toward the center line of the body.

Figure 4: Bring the right heel onto the floor, with the weight coming to rest squarely on the heel. It may feel like your weight is now on the outside of the foot. Compare the appearance of the right and left leg as well as how they feel.

Repeat on the left side.

The scooped feet on the left resemble the 86-year old feet on the right. Both resemble feet of young children.

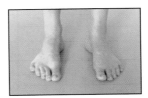
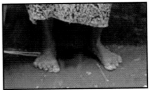

EXPLORATION #12 BREATHING FREE

This simple exercise will demonstrate the relationship between abdominal muscles and breathing.

- Tense the muscles of your abdomen as though you were tightening a corset or closing a pull-string purse. Your navel is drawing inward towards your spine. Continue to hold these muscles tight as you ask yourself the following questions:

    – Is my breathing free and relaxed?

    – Does my torso feel open and spacious or contracted and tight?

    – Is my spine elongated or compressed?

    – Is the rest of my body—my neck and jaw, my chest, shoulders and back—relaxed or tense?

- Now slowly release the abdominal muscles and notice how the answer to each one of these questions changes. This is because your diaphragm is no longer restricted. This greater sense of relaxation is only possible when abdominal muscles are relaxed.

Relaxing the belly is at the heart of natural breathing. Without a relaxed belly, the diaphragm is engaged in a way that restricts its free and easy movement.

Aligning the bones is also at the heart of natural breathing. Without aligned bones, muscles are forced into chronic contraction, thus restricting our ability to breathe easily.

LET GO TO BREATHE

Everyone breathes all the time without having to think about it, so why all the fuss about how one breathes? An earlier chapter on breathing made the point that breathing is more than just an exchange of oxygen and carbon dioxide. The way we breathe can contribute in a big way to our overall health and well-being.

Conscious breathing, which tends to be deeper and lower in the belly is different from automatic, unconscious breathing, which tends to be shallow and higher in the chest. How you breathe is as important as anything (even natural alignment!) in determining your state of health and state of mind.

Perhaps the simplest and most effective way to address breathing is to do nothing at all other than to observe it. Instead of trying to control or manage the breath in any way, remove yourself from being in charge and simply notice what happens when you relax and let go.

Relaxing and letting go allows the physical center of gravity to drop into the abdomen. When this happens, each breath is naturally born from deep within the belly, then fills the belly and the back, and then drops away again. Align the bones. Relax all tension. Let go. By simply creating the conditions that are conducive to natural breathing, breathing happens.

Don't try to hurry any change. That, alone, will undermine it. Change happens on its own when you set your intention and practice letting go as often as you can remember. The rest will take care of itself.

PART III

Putting It All Together

Think with the whole body.

Taisen Deshimaru

DOWN TO BASICS
Sitting, Standing, Bending, Walking and Sleeping

Putting it all together is what this is all about. By learning how to sit, stand, bend, walk and sleep, you will have the tools to practice and apply these principles of natural alignment all day long in every situation in which you find yourself.

This is never easy at first. One of the biggest stumbling blocks is simply remembering to do this, not just once but over and over again. The more often you notice how you are sitting at the computer, or bending over to tie your shoe, or walking from your car into the grocery store, the more you will reinforce new habits that gradually build upon themselves. Think of simple ways to remind yourself—a chime that sounds on your computer, sticky notes on your refrigerator door or bathroom mirror, a rubber band around your wrist. Do whatever it takes to trigger yourself to remember to pay attention. It is important that every time you remember any aspect of this information, you apply it as best you know how.

Practicing awareness of the body in this way is like putting money into a savings account. The new habits build on themselves and the earnings become exponential. Eventually, you will be surprised to find how often you are aware of yourself as a body, not just a mental process. At this point, big changes are occurring, changes that are aiding your overall health and sense of well-being.

HOW TO SIT

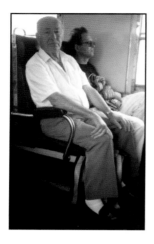 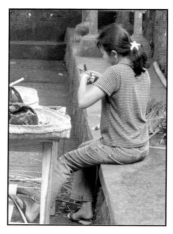 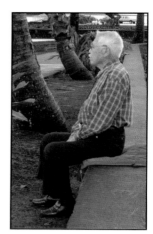

- Establish your SOLID SEAT (Exploration #4). You may want to sit on a wedge. (See Appendix).

- Relax the belly.

- Release the front of your chest downward as your back rises up behind you.

- Roll one shoulder, then the other onto the top of the rib cage.

- Drop your chin towards your chest, then slowly roll it up the front of your throat, releasing any tension as you do this.

- Look forward using your eyes.

- Breathe in a natural way.

SITTING SHORTCUT

– Sit on your sit bones.
– Relax your belly.
– Release your chest down.
– Do shoulder rolls.

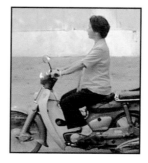 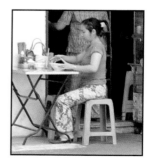

HOW TO STAND

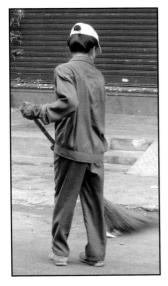
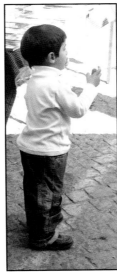
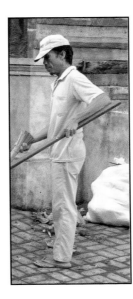
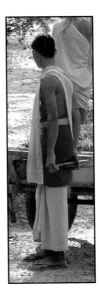

- Stand with heels six inches apart and toes eight inches apart. Knees are straight but not locked.

- Bow slightly at the hips until you can see your ankles.

- Relax the belly.

- Release the chest down.

- Roll one shoulder at a time onto the top of the rib cage.

- Drop your chin slightly, and roll it up the front of the throat, continuously relaxing any tension that arises. Do not let this change any of the adjustments you have already made.

- Breathe in a natural and relaxed way.

> ## STANDING SHORTCUT
>
> – Look down at your ankles, and relax your belly.
> – Lift your face enough to see out in front of you.
> – Relax.

HOW TO WALK

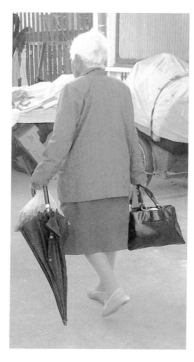 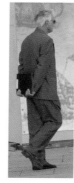 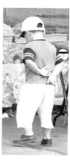 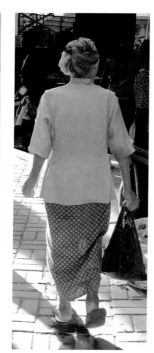

- Bow slightly at the hips and lean forward.

- The top of your head leads you forward as you step onto your left foot.

- As the weight comes onto the left leg, the left knee bends in a slight lunge. The knees are aimed toward the little toes.

- Repeat as you step onto the right leg, with the head leading and the right knee bending slightly as the weight lands on the right leg.

- Use your eyes to look up instead of lifting your chin.

WALKING SHORTCUT

– Lean forward from the hips.
– Your knee bends slightly as the leg receives your weight.

HOW TO SIT FOR MEDITATION

- Establish your SOLID SEAT (Exploration #4) on a cushion or chair, letting the pelvis have weight.

- Relax your belly, experiencing your center of gravity in the abdomen.

- Release the chest down, as the midback rises up and opens out behind you.

- Roll one shoulder at a time onto the top of the rib cage.

- Drop the chin, and slide it slowly up the throat, lengthening the neck and relaxing all tension. Chest stays down.

- Let the inner body (the skeleton) support you so that the outer body (everything else) relaxes.

- Observe the breath rising and falling in a natural way.

> **When it comes to meditating, there are no shortcuts to being mindful of the body and its alignment.**

SLEEPING AND RESTING ON YOUR BACK

- Lying flat on the floor rolls the rib cage backward and causes the lower back to arch. This can interfere with one's ability to fully relax. Supporting the head and shoulders with two soft pillows takes the arch out of the lumbar spine and makes it possible to relax.

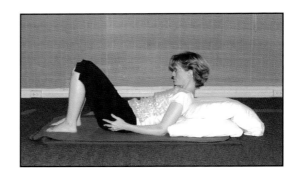

- Lie down with two pillows positioned so that one pillow comes to the bottom edge of the shoulder blades, and the other pillow just under the top edge of the shoulders.

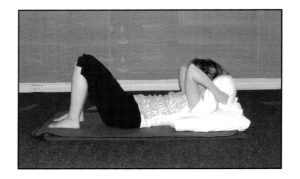

- Press into the floor with both elbows, and 'hitch' the middle of your back up toward your head (rolling the rib cage wheel forward).

- Reach up with both hands on either side of the top pillow and roll under the top pillow so that your head is supported with the chin dropped slightly and the back of your neck long (head wheel rolling forward).

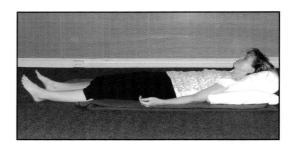

- Observe the breath, and let all tension drop away.

LYING ON YOUR SIDE

- Lie on your side with one or two pillows under your head. Bend your knees slightly.

- Bring the pillow(s) up to your shoulder, so that the neck is fully supported.

- Press into the floor with the hand of the upper arm, and move the pubic bone out behind you several inches (Figure A).

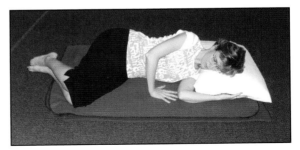

Figure A

- Draw the pillow, along with your head and shoulders, toward your knees. Feel your lower back release as the spine lengthens (Figure B).

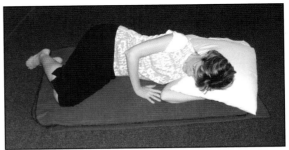

Figure B

- Bring your left arm to rest along your left side (Figure C).

- Knees stay together, although feet can be apart. You may place a pillow between your knees if you like.

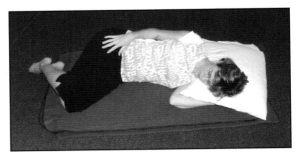

Figure C

- Back your head up slightly, tucking your chin to lengthen the back of the neck.

NOTE: You might feel as though you are curling into a round ball. You actually have extended your spine.

A FEW PARTING THOUGHTS

- Don't try too hard. Relax and trust.

- Nevertheless, keep practicing as often as you can remember.

- Apply the mind to the body using passive verbs (rise, drop, sink) instead of active verbs (push, pull, lift).

- Let your pelvis have weight. Drop roots into the earth. Be grounded.

- Think length through your spine with space between the vertebrae, equal in the front and the back.

- Think openness and freedom in your joints.

- Feel boundaries melting. Feel inner and outer merging.

- Let the breath be low, soft and quiet. Experience it in your back more than in your front.

- Relax your jaw and neck and drop your chin.

- When in doubt—about anything—relax your belly.

- Smile.

LIST OF ILLUSTRATIONS

ENDNOTES

AUTHOR'S NOTES

Kendra Ing deserves credit for astute insights and thought-provoking discussions that were pivotal to these comments.

INTRODUCTION

Pages 1-2

Kalb, Claudia, ed. "The Great Back Debate." Newsweek. 26 April 2004.
Spinal fusion surgery statistics and epidural injections.

Page 2

Staehler, Rick, M.D. "What Are Potential Risks and Side Effects of Epidural Steroid Injection?" Spine-Health.com, August 2000, http://www.spinehealth.com/topics/conserv/epidural/feature/ep06.html

CHAPER 1 THE SHAPE WE'RE IN

Page 3

Most research involving the incidence of musculoskeletal pain in various populations compares statistics among Western countries. Much of the evidence outside of the Western world is anecdotal and relates to observations of how people live, work and age. However, what few studies have been conducted corroborate these observations, as follows:

A.D.A.M. Healthcare Center. http://adam.about.com/reports/000035_4.htm
Even in the U.S, the rate of osteoarthritis is geographical. Although the average rate of osteoarthritis among older adults in the U.S. is 60%, it can vary widely in certain geographical

regions. In the U.S., the rates in older adults are lowest (34%) in Hawaii and highest (70.3%) in Alabama. In general, the highest prevalence of arthritis in America occurs in the central and northwestern states.

Brooks, Peter. "Inflammation as an Important Feature of Osteoarthritis." Bulletin of the World Health Organization, 81:9, Sept. 2003, pp. 689-690.

Regional differences are evident in a pattern of osteoarthritis across the world, with hip osteoarthritis being less common in Africa and Asia than in Western countries.

Khataev, Nikolai, M.D., Ph.D. "The Burden of Musculoskeletal Conditions at the Start of the New Millennium." World Health Organization, Report of a WHO Scientific Group. WHO Technical Report Series Number 919,2003. www.who.int/entity/bulletin/volumes/81/9/en/PHC.pdf.

This article states that musculoskeletal and other noncommunicable diseases account for the largest share of the burden in the developed world, while communicable diseases continue to be the primary health issue in the developing world.

Rottensten, Kirsten. "Division of Aging and Seniors." Chronic Diseases in Canada. Canada: Population Health Directorate, Health Promotion and Programs Branch, 17:3, 1996, www.phac-aspc.gc.ca/publicat/cdic-mcc/17-3/b_e.html

From their comparison between Japanese-Oriental and American-white subjects, as well as subjects from other population studies, Hoaglund et al. concluded that primary hip osteoarthritis is a disorder of European-American whites. This is supported by the low rates of hip osteoarthritis among black populations from Jamaica, South Africa, Nigeria and Liberia in contrast to the higher rates of hip osteoarthritis among populations from North England, West Germany, Czechoslovakia and Switzerland.

Page 5

Kalb, Claudia, ed. "The Great Back Debate." Newsweek. 26 April 2004.

Discussion of incidence of back pain in America and the costs incurred for treating this condition.

Pages 8-9

Modern times have led to a more casual, "relaxed" style of living. This raises the question: Are we really more relaxed? We tend to equate less formality with being more relaxed. While less formal attire may indeed contribute to feeling more relaxed, slouching and more casual ways of inhabiting our bodies generate tension in muscles and stress to the nervous system, thereby opposing an ability to genuinely relax.

CHAPTER 2: DESIGN FOR LIFE

Page 16

Olshansky, S. Jay, Bruce A. Carnes, and Robert N. Butler. "If Humans Were Built to Last," Scientific American, March 2001, pp 51-55.

This article speculates that humans have evolved badly, leaving us to age with a whole host of degenerative problems, many related to our structural design. The suggestion is made that back pain is the inevitable outcome of a flawed adaptive process as we evolved from our quadripedal ancestry, which has resulted in spines that are not designed well for our current bipedal reality. When we look more closely at those people who age without the litany of modern, degenerative problems, it becomes evident that evolution, which by definition is a work in progress and therefore can never be "wrong," has designed a human spine that is a masterpiece of architectural wonder. Perhaps the whole quarrel between evolutionists and creationists might be resolved by looking beyond the intractable either/or stances and adopting a both/and view that considers that evolution might be the way an unfathomable intelligent design expresses itself.

Page 17

There is a common assumption that people who carry heavy loads on their heads typically suffer injury and degeneration of the spine. This is certainly true in cases where people have misaligned skeletons to begin with. Only those people who easily maintain naturally aligned balance should ever carry loads on their heads. Any study in this area must be undertaken by researchers who fully understand the details of natural alignment. Otherwise, the results will be meaningless. This author met a lively 103-year old woman in Indonesia who, according to her granddaughter, carried river rocks on her head for decades. Asked if she had ever suffered back pain as a result, the woman answered, "No."

Page 18

A central axis is a line around which a geometric figure rotates. It appears conceptually in mathematics, engineering and biology. This concept replicates itself in the boundless universe in the rotations of planets as well as the infinitesimal level where the DNA ladders spiral around a central axis. An axis typifies a concept of organization and symmetry, of stability and return.

CHAPTER 3: AMAZING GRACE

People who maintain natural alignment into old age are living treasures who hold secrets of healthy, relaxed living in aligned bodies. Because they have never lost what they instinctively knew as young children, they are unaware of how unique they are. As these people die, there will be fewer and fewer people who will be the keepers of this innate understanding. The task of parents and teachers will be to support young children in remaining natural—not an easy thing to manage, when there are so few examples and role models for them.

CHAPTER 4: ARCHITECTURE IN FLESH AND BONE

Page 32

Zome™ Toy. Zome is a Registered Trademark of Zometool, Inc., 601 E. 48th Ave., Denver, CO 80216 USA; Zometool.com

R. Buckminster Fuller (1895-1983) invented the geodesic dome and first described tensegrity—a contraction of tensional integrity—as a structural-relationship principle. According to Timothy Wilkin, M.D., www.synearth.net/TensegrityHtml/Tensegrity/html, "The forces between the bones and muscles are held in constant balance, with the muscle providing continuous pull and the bones discontinuous push. Tensegrity is the pattern that results when push and pull have a win-win relationship with each other (emphasis added). Push and pull seem so common and ordinary in our experience of life that we humans think little of these forces. Most of us assume they are simple opposites. In and out. Back and forth. Force directed in one direction or its opposite. Fuller explained that these fundamental phenomena were not opposites, but complements that could always be found together."

Page 35

Lujan, Barbara F., and Ronald J. White. Human Physiology in Space. National Space Biomedical Research Institute, www.nsbri.org/HumanPhysSpace/focus6/ep_development. html

This site offers a concise description of the components and function of bones.

Todd, Mabel E. The Thinking Body. Hightstown, NJ: Princeton Book Company, 1937, pp.59-60.

Page 36

Bamboo scaffolding is commonly used throughout Asia, even in the construction of multi-story, high-rise buildings. The secret to the stability of this scaffolding is the integrity of the verticality of the foundation posts along with stable joints that lash the horizontal cross poles to the vertical posts.

Page 40

McClintic, Robert J. Basic Anatomy and Physiology of the Human Body. New York: John Wiley and Sons, 1980, pp. 157-160.

Page 46
French, A. P. Newtonian Physics, M.I.T. Series. New York: W. W. Norton and Company, 1971, pp. 123-124.

Page 47
So far, the information regarding the angle of the sacrum has received little scientific attention in terms of what is natural. However, there is anecdotal information based on the x-rays of an older Portuguese man whose spine appears to be naturally aligned and who, not coincidentally, can easily carry heavy pails of fish on his head. Information such as this raises many questions regarding the natural arch at the base of the spine. What is the angle of the ceiling of the sacrum (sacral platform) in healthy babies just learning to walk? What is this angle in healthy adults who spend their entire lives in natural alignment? What about the natural shapes of the lumbar vertebrae and intervertebral discs? Does this change in some people as they go out of alignment? While there seems to be no data relating to what is natural in this regard, any future study of spines of aligned people versus people who are not aligned promises to reveal many interesting insights.

Page 49
Ebersberger, Ingo, Dirk Metzler, Carsten Schwarz, and Svante Pääbo. "Genomewide Comparison of DNA Sequences between Humans and Chimpanzees." American Journal of Human Genetics. 70:1490-1497, 2002.
The ability to brachiate—to move by swinging from the arms from one hand hold to another—only occurs in some apes and spider monkeys.

Pages 54-56
McClintic, Robert J. Basic Anatomy and Physiology of the Human Body. New York: John Wiley and Sons, 1980, pp. 291-301.

CHAPTER 5: THREE WHEELS OF ALIGNMENT
Page 63
There are a number of painful conditions that fall under the category of chronic pelvic pain syndrome (CPPS)—prostatitis, interstitial cystitis, pelvic floor myalgia, incontinence—all of which in one way or another involve the muscles of the pelvic floor. The pelvic floor muscles consist of the levator ani muscles, which go between the pubis and the sacrum; in women, a central group of these muscles surrounds the urethra, the vagina and the rectum. Beneath this floor, there are also sphincter muscles around the anus and urethra. The obterator internus muscles and the pirisormyusformus muscles control the

movement of the hip; but because they insert on the pubic bone, they also can have some effect on the urethra. The pudendal nerve supports the muscles of the pelvic floor. Overall, these muscle groups serve functions of support of the internal organs, act as sphincters for the bladder and are involved in sexual function. Interestingly, recent developments in treatments of the above-listed conditions that have been particularly successful are related to teaching patients how to relax the pelvic floor. This is particularly noteworthy because the cause of all of these conditions remains largely unknown, although it is not unreasonable to suppose that unnatural placement of the pelvic bone might detrimentally affect what would otherwise be a symmetrical arrangement of these muscles' fibers.

Hetrick, Diane C., et al. "Musculoskeletal Dysfunction in Men with Chronic Pelvic Pain Syndrome Type III: A Case-control Study." Journal of Urology. 170(3):828-831, September 2003.

In a comparison of men with and without pelvic pain, those with pain had significantly greater tension in pelvic floor muscles.

True, Lawrence, et al. "Prostate Histopathology and Chronic Prostatitis/Chronic Pelvic Pain Syndrome: A Prospective Biopsy Study." Journal of Urology. 162(11):2014, December 1999.

The term prostatitis means inflammation of the prostate, which has been the primary diagnosis of men presenting chronic pelvic pain. This study reveals that only 5% of patients complaining of chronic pain showed moderate to severe prostate inflammation, raising the question of whether numerous cases of prostatitis might be more accurately diagnosed as chronic tension in pelvic floor muscles. An examination of the posture of men who present with these symptoms might well reveal the cause, in some cases, to be the tilt of the pelvis.

Weiss, Jerome M., M.D., Associate Clinical Professor, University of California, San Francisco; founder, Pacific Center for Pelvic Pain and Dysfunction. Interstitial Cystitis Network, Chat Log (© 1999, www.ic-network.com)

Dr. Weiss suggests that pelvic pain is caused by repetitive, sustained or severe overload of the muscles of the pelvic floor. "Through various life experiences, there can be an increasing degree of tension that eventually causes the symptoms to develop. Some of these are holding patterns and tensions in the bladder floor that develops at an early age. This can be the result of sexual abuse or traumatic toilet training and even dance or gymnastic training that teaches children to hold tight those muscles, repetitive minor trauma, straining to have a bowel an accident, or fall, or sports injury …When humans are stressed, the coccyx pulls forward. When it pulls forward, it compresses the organs that run through those muscles and pulls them up against the pubic bone. Successful treatment programs sometimes include postural re-education and application of relaxation techniques."

Wise, David, Ph.D., and Rodney Anderson, M.D. Headache in the Pelvis: A New

Understanding and Treatment for Prostatitis and Chronic Pelvic Pain Syndromes. COP: National Center for Pelvic Pain, 2005.

CPPS is often caused by overuse of pelvic muscles, as if trying "to protect the genitals, rectum and contents of the pelvis from injury or pain by contracting the pelvic muscles. This tendency becomes exaggerated in predisposed individuals and over time results in pelvic pain and dysfunction." Dr. Wise suggests that the reason prostatitis is largely resistant to treatment is because some patients chronically (and, of course, unknowingly) contract their pelvic floor muscles, giving irritated tissues little or no chance to heal. This in turn can lead to symptoms commonly associated with prostatitis. Progressive relaxation techniques to break the cycle of "shortened pelvic muscles and connective tissue" are the treatment commonly used by Dr. Wise and his Stanford University colleagues at the Prostatitis Foundation.

Page 65

Reports of how much the human head weighs vary from 8-15 pounds. A compromise would have the average adult head weighing approximately 11.5 pounds.

CHAPTER 6: BREATHING LIFE INTO STRUCTURE

Page 68

Evans, D. W., M.D.,and L. C. Lum, M.D. "Hyperventilation: An Important Cause of Pseudo-angina." Lancet, 1(8004):155-7, January 1977.

Magarian, Gregory J., M.D., Deborah A. Middaugh, M.D., and Douglas H. Linz, M.D. "Hyperventilation Syndrome: A Diagnosis Begging for Recognition." Western Journal of Medicine. 138(5):733-736, May 1983.

Hyperventilation syndrome is usually associated with emotional triggers and thoracic breathing tendency. "Among the most difficult and frustrating patients for physicians are those with multiple complaints involving many organ systems who, despite seeing numerous physicians, fail to obtain a satisfactory explanation or relief from their symptoms. They often have a 'positive review of systems.' After numerous physicians have been seen and multiple diagnostic tests have been done, which have excluded organic disorders, such patients are often dismissed as having nothing wrong with them or having a severe neurosis, anxiety, depression, hypochondriasis or hysteria, despite the persistence of symptoms that may be disabling in their work and other aspects of everyday living. Unfortunately, this scenario continues to be a common occurrence and is the frequent setting in which the hyperventilation syndrome is recognized, months or years after its onset....Long-term control may be achieved by relaxation therapy and retraining patients to become diaphragmatic rather than thoracic breathers." These doctors are on the right track. Breathing well is vital. So is natural alignment of the skeleton, which makes efficient breathing possible.

Magarian, Gregory J., M.D. "Hyperventilation Syndrome: Infrequently Recognized Common Expressions of Anxiety and Stress." Medicine. 61, June 1982, 219-236.

www.iscid.org/encyclopedia/Bohr_Effect

The Bohr Effect is an adaptation in animals to release oxygen in oxygen-starved tissues in capillaries where respiratory carbon dioxide lowers blood pH. It was first described by the Danish physiologist Christian Bohr in 1904. Normal breathing keeps hemoglobin, the principle carrier of oxygen to the body, saturated with oxygen (O_2). When we breathe more than is necessary (hyperventilation), we lose CO_2 that is essential for O_2 utilization. Ironically, the more one breathes, the less oxygen becomes available to the tissues of the body. In terms of breathing, more is not necessarily a good thing. Instructions to breathe deeply when under stress or during a panic attack can make things worse. The combined causes of panic attacks—stress, habitual over-breathing and catastrophic thinking—all build upon each other, sometimes even mimicking symptoms of a heart attack. A distinction needs to be made between deep breathing and "over-breathing" (commonly and mistakenly thought of as deep breathing), which underutilizes the action of the diaphragm and interferes with the body's ability to use oxygen. Actual deep breathing is low and relaxed, the result of elastic movement of the diaphragm. This kind of breathing is soft, quiet, nourishing and "deep" in the belly.

Pages 62-63
Todd, Mabel E. The Thinking Body. Hightstown, NJ: Princeton Book Company, 1937, p.234.

Pages 64-65
Koch, Liz. The Psoas Book. Felton, CA: Guinea Pig Publications, 1997.

CHAPTER 7: MEET YOUR FEET

Page 80
McClintic, Robert J. Basic Anatomy and Physiology of the Human Body. New York: John Wiley and Sons, 1980, pp. 157-160.

Page 81
Rao, Udaya Bhaskara and Benjamin Joseph. "The Influence of Footwear on the Prevalence of Flat Foot." The Journal of Bone and Joint Surgery. 74B(4):525-527, 1992.

This study of 2300 children determined that flat foot was most common in children who wore close-toed shoes, less common in those who wore slippers or sandals and least common in those who went barefoot. The study concluded that shoe-wearing in early childhood is detrimental to the development of a normal longitudinal arch.

CHAPTER 8: PREGNANT WITH POSSIBILITIES

Pages 76-82

Gaskin, Ina May. Ina May's Guide to Childbirth. New York: Bantam, 2003.

Goer, Henci. The Thinking Woman's Guide to a Better Birth. New York: Berkley Publishing Group, 1999.

McCutheon, Susan. Natural Childbirth the Bradley Way. New York: Bantam Book, 1984.

CHAPTER 9: OUR CHILDREN IN PERIL

Pages 94-95

Gorman, Christine. "Why More Kids Are Getting Hurt." Time Magazine. 6 June 2005.

Pediatric orthopedic surgery is a recent and growing specialty. Doctors say they are treating types of injuries never before seen in people so young. They chalk it up to overtraining, but could it also be our changing habits of use?

CHAPTER 10: WORKING OUT OR WORKING IN?

Page 98

"Common Sports Injuries." Merck Manual of Diagnosis and Therapy, Section 5, Chapter 62. Rahway, NJ: Merck Publishing, 2004.

"More than ten million sports injuries are treated each year in the USA. Athletes and nonathletes share many similar injuries. For example, lateral and medial epicondylitis (tennis elbow) can be caused by carrying a suitcase, turning a screwdriver or opening a stuck door; and patellofemoral pain (runner's knee) can be caused by excessive pronation while walking."

www.americansportsdata.com/sports_injury1.asp

Health club membership rose 266% between 1987 and 2001. With it, there has been a corresponding jump in injuries.

Pages 98-99

Endorphins and the high one gets from some types of exercise has an up side and a down side. The down side becomes evident in those cases where people must exercise in order to feel good, happy, comfortable. Some people become highly agitated and feel like they will jump out of their skins if their exercise routines are interrupted for any period of time. This indicates autonomic nervous system dysfunction that could potentially be the result of excessive exercise.

Brene, Stefan. The Journal of Neuroscience. 22(18):8133-8138. 15 September 2002.

"Although speculative, the increasing knowledge about FosB suggests that it, or the various molecular pathways it regulates, could be a suitable target for the development of pharmacological treatments for a range of disorders…(including) eating disorders, pathological gambling, excessive exercise…."

Pert, Candace B. Molecules of Emotion: The Science Behind Mind-Body Medicine. New York: Scribner, 1997.

Pert is a pioneer in the field of neuropeptide research, having discovered opiate receptors and contributed to the recognition in the scientific community of the mind-body connection. This book makes this complicated subject easy to understand.

Werme, Martin, Peter Thoren, Lars Olson, and Stefan Brene. "Running and Cocaine Both Upregulate Dynorphin mRNA in Medial Caudate Putamen." European Journal of Neuroscience. 12:8, August 2000, p. 2967.

According to these neuroscientists, "Physical activities such as long-distance running can be habit-forming and associated with a sense of well-being to a degree that justifies comparison with drug-induced addictive behaviours."

Page 101

Todd, Mabel E. The Thinking Body. Hightstown, NJ: Princeton Book Company, 1937, p. 40.

Page 106

Naturally aligned athletes who have reached the top of their sport include Olympic runner Carl Lewis, basketball player Yao Ming, tennis player Venus Williams, football player Jerry Rice, baseball player Roberto Clemente and a disproportionate number of runners from Kenya, among others. These people illustrate the innate strength and freedom of movement available to those who inhabit their bodies in a natural way.

CHAPTER 11: IMPLICATIONS FOR HEALTH

Page 112

Osteoarthritis. National Institute of Health, National Institute of Arthritis and Musculoskeltal Symptoms. www.niams.nih.gov/hi/topics/arthritis/oahandout.htm

Page 114

Bone Health and Osteoporosis: A Report of the Surgeon General. October 2004, www.surgeongeneral.gov/library/bonehealth

Brown, Susan E., Ph.D., Better Bones, Better Body: Beyond Estrogen and Calcium. Los Angeles, CA: Keats Publishing, 2000.

This book offers a wealth of information related to osteoporosis.

Report, "Osteoporosis Management." The Online Series of Continuing Medical Education, American Medical Association. www.ama-assn.org/ama/pub/category/2797.html

Overview of osteoporosis and recommended treatments.

Page 116

www.ars.usda.gov/is/AR/archive/mar03/osteo0303.htm

The cause of osteoporosis remains largely unknown.

Alexander, F. M. The Essential Writings of F. Matthias Alexander: The Alexander Technique. Edward Maisel, ed. Secaucus, NJ: Carol Publishing Group, 1990.

"There is hardly a bodily function, from digestion to respiration, which cannot be gravely interfered with by faulty bodily coordination."

Pages 116-117

Misalignment of bones causes tension in muscles. Tension in muscles restricts free, relaxed breathing. And free, relaxed breathing is necessary for the parasympathetic nervous system (the relaxation response) to be engaged. When the relaxation response is not engaged, the sympathetic nervous system dominates, and stress and anxiety, tension and pain, and ultimately dysfunction and disease can be the result. Comparing the overall health of people who have always lived with naturally aligned bones against those who have not is likely to be very revealing. So far, such a study has never been done.

CHAPTER 12: BEYOND THE PHYSICAL

It is in the fields of psychology and spirituality that the most innovative and far-reaching approaches to the body-mind are taking place. From addressing symptoms of dysfunction and distress to elevated states of consciousness, the individual is seen as an integrated whole and a system of interdependent parts that reflect an inner and outer reality. In a gradually developing process of understanding how this works, there have been many pioneers who have built upon each other's discoveries to further our comprehension of what turns out to have been described by spiritual teachers through the ages—the ability to relax mentally and physically are interdependent upon each other and lie at the heart of experiencing inner peace.

Hans Selye was the first in the modern medical profession to confirm the influence of stress on people's ability to cope with life's many challenges. Herbert Benson defined the relaxation response and was one of the first doctors to bring spirituality and healing into medicine. Candace Pert's research shed light on how the body-mind functions as a single psychosomatic network of information molecules that control one's health and physiology. Jon Kabat-Zinn brought practices of mindfulness meditation into mainstream medicine and showed how the practice of mindfulness can address a wide spectrum of health issues by reducing stress. Had these people not been willing to study themselves as closely as many other scientists observe external phenomena, their work would have been meaningless. This is the opportunity each one of us has—to be self-studying scientists by turning our attention inside and discovering for ourselves who we really are.

Page 124

Agazarian, Y. Systems-Centered Therapy for Groups. New York and London: Guilford Press, 1997.

Begin, A.. E., and S. L. Garfield, (eds.). Handbook of Psychotherapy and Behavior Change (4th Ed.). New York: John Wiley and Sons, 1994, p. 238.

James, W. "A Study of the Expression of Bodily Posture." Journal of General Psychology. 7, 1932, pp. 405-406.

Rossberg-Gempton, I., and G. Poole. The Effect of Open and Closed Postures. COP, 1993.

Sikes, Charlotte, and John Westefeld. "Therapists' Postures: Response to Spinal Alignment." JASNH. University of Iowa: Reysen Group, 1:4, 1539-8714, 2002, pp. 57–68. www.jasnh.com/a9.htm

This article, quoted in part below, is a compendium of other articles and studies that detail observable insights into the mental and emotional details that are observable, consciously or otherwise, by how we inhabit our bodies:

"This study examines how a therapist's spinal alignment, defined as the organization of the three primary body weights (the skull, thorax, and pelvis) around a vertical plumbline, affects clients' perceptions of themselves. (One) study showed that open postures were associated with increased positive emotions, whereas closed postures elicited negative emotions (Rossberg-Gempton et al., 1992). Because of the effect posture may have on emotion, and because studies show that high distress levels in therapists may prevent the growth of clients, or even lead to negative changes in them, a therapist's posture may indirectly affect therapeutic outcome (Begin and Garfield, 1994). According to Begin and Garfield (1994), the well-being and adjustment of the therapist plays a role in optimal therapeutic results. These effects of posture relate to 'postures as felt,' a term which refers to the experience of a posture (James,

1890). 'Postures as seen,' in contrast, relates to the observation of postures (James, 1890). These terms are useful because postures appear to affect both the one assuming the posture, and those observing him or her. Something as subtle as integrated body movements, judged by Posture-Gesture Mergers (PGMs), corresponds with more truthful and relaxed verbal communication (Winter, 1989)....Showing that postures do not just reflect internal states, but can produce them, Riskind and Gotay (1982) found that tasks designed to cause learned helplessness were more effective when performed by people in slouched spinal positions than erect spinal positions....In addition, muscle relaxation has been shown to decrease or alleviate anxiety and guilt feelings (Laird, 1984; Rasid and Parish, 1998)....Systems-Centered Psychotherapy (SCT), a technique growing in popularity among therapists in the last ten years, requires therapists and clients both to sit 'centered,' which is defined as sitting up straight, over one's sit bones (the part of the pelvis one can feel on the chair or floor when sitting up straight) with one's feet planted on the ground (Agazarian, 1997). SCT theory holds that in addition to decreasing anxiety and tension, an erect but relaxed, posture provides clients more energy to put toward therapeutic exploration (Agazarian, 1997). In support of this theory, one medical study found that participants going from erect to slouched postures uniformly decreased in their principal resonance frequency (Kitazaki, 1998). Results suggest that spinal alignment affects the vibrational level of the body."

Tolle, Eckhart. The Power of Now. New World Library: 1999, pp. 94-100.

Winter, D., C. Widell, G. Truitt, and J. George-Falvey. "Empirical Studies of Posture-Gesture Mergers." Journal of Nonverbal Behavior. 1989, pp. 207-222.

APPENDIX

This directory is not intended to exclude any modality or organization that is compatible with the principles of natural alignment. This brief listing points to a possible starting point for locating a teacher in your area.

Natural Alignment

The principles and guidelines that are taught at the Balance Center inspired the writing of this book. Here you will find all the hands-on, one-on-one help you need to learn how to put this into practice. The Balance Center offers ongoing classes (including yoga in Balance), workshops, intensives and private sessions. It is enormously helpful (in most cases, essential) to have the hands-on experience of working with a teacher who can help guide you to a place of natural alignment that unconscious muscle patterns might otherwise prevent. Balance is especially helpful for anyone in pain, although anyone can learn to feel more comfortable and relaxed by learning how to inhabit the body in a natural way. There are 25-30 trained Balance teachers throughout the country. Call the Balance Center to find out if there is one in your area. Teacher training is also available.

The Balance Center
560 Oxford Avenue
Palo Alto, CA 94306
(650) 856-2000
Jean Couch, Director
www.balancecenter.com
info@balancecenter.com

Classes, workshops and private sessions in natural alignment and how to sit, stand, bend, walk and generally inhabit your body in a natural, relaxed and comfortable way. Once learned, these principles can be applied to exercising and playing sports, working in the garden, sitting at the computer and all other daily activities. Kathleen is periodically available to travel to conduct workshops and give presentations.

Wellspring Center for Natural Alignment
190 Kamehameha Avenue, Room 5
Hilo, HI 96720
(808) 896-4629
Kathleen Porter
www.agelessspine.com
contact@agelessspine.com

Complimentary Modalities

Alexander Technique, developed by F. M. Alexander over a century ago, has helped thousands of people learn how to inhabit their bodies in a more natural, relaxed way. Alexander Technique places important emphasis on awareness and conscious release of unhelpful habits. While certain differences exist between the guidelines of AT and the from-the-ground-up approach of Balance as developed by Jean Couch, the similarities are meaningful. Studying with a well-trained, sensitive Alexander Technique teacher can help set anyone on the path to becoming his or her own best teacher, the ultimate goal of any one of these approaches.

Alexander Alliance
2967 Schoolhouse Lane, Apt. 306
Philadelphia, PA 19144
Martha and Bruce Fertman, Directors
(215) 844-0670
www.alexanderalliance.com
contact@alexanderalliance.com

American Society for the Alexander Technique
P.O. Box 60008
Florence, MA 01062
(800) 473-0620 or (413) 584-2359
www.alexandertech.org
info@amsat.ws

Bodywork, Acupuncture and Such

Rolfing, Massage, Acupuncture, Reiki, Healing Touch, Cranial-Sacral Therapy

Anyone who has experienced hands-on work of this sort knows that bodyworkers, energy healers and acupuncturists perform an important service that benefits countless people. Some practitioners have a particular gift for facilitating a process of healing by skillfully creating conditions for energy to flow more easily. Remember, healing is an inside job. Others can only help you. It is useful to think of the therapist as your assistant in this process, with you as the active participant who chooses to let go of whatever it is you no longer need. Be patient with yourself. Align your bones as best you know how, bring attention to the breath and the present moment as often as you can remember, then draw on the help of others to support and encourage you in this process.

The best way to find the right practitioner can be to ask others for a recommendation. Word-of-mouth can be very reliable. Ultimately, your own instincts and experiences will be the most important factors in making a choice. Some practitioners, such as those for massage and acupuncture, are licensed by regional boards; others are certified through national organizations such as those listed below. Some of those listed below combine bodywork with movement.

Rolf Institute of Structural Integration
5055 Chaparral Court, Suite 103
Boulder, CO 80301
(800) 530-8875 or (303) 449-5903
www.rolf.org
info@rolf.org

The Upledger Institute (Cranial-Sacral Therapy)
11211 Prosperity Farms Road, Suite D-325
Palm Beach Gardens, FL 33410
(561) 622-4334
www.upledger.com
upledger@upledger.com

Healing Touch International
445 Union Blvd., Suite 105
Lakewood, CO 80228
(303) 989-7982
Fax (303) 980-8683

www.healingtouch.net
HTIheal@aol.com
Hanna Somatic Education
605 Calle de Valdes
Santa Fe, NM 87505
(505) 699-8284
www.somatics.com
inquiry@somatics.com

Aston Enterprises (Aston Patterning)
P.O. Box 3568
Incline Village, NV 89450
(775) 831-8228
www.astonenterprises.com
info@astonenterprises.com

The Zero Balancing Association
8640 Guilford Road, Suite 240
Columbia, MD 21046
(410) 381-8956
www.zerobalancing.com

Hellerwork Structural Integration
www.hellerwork.com
info@hellerwork.com

Movement, Exercise & Martial Arts

Qi Qong, Tai Chi, Yoga, Feldenkrais, Aikido, Kendo

These disciplines have a lot to offer when practiced in a way that reinforces the understanding that true relaxation in any activity is the cornerstone of good health. If possible, choose those forms of exercise, and the teachers who teach them, that promote and encourage natural alignment of the bones and an innate strength that is simply a byproduct of being structurally aligned. Notice if your motivation for participating in any of these activities is driven by a wish to build strength in muscles, stretch away tension or by a concern about how you look more than how you feel. Ask around in your community and try out different classes until you find what best supports alignment and relaxation in all activities.

Breathing Resources

Anything that helps you to align your bones and relax more deeply will enhance breathing. This is important because nothing is more important in terms of health and overall well-being than natural, relaxed breathing. Letting go of tension in order to breathe more naturally takes time and practice. Keep tuning in to the breath in as many moments of each day as you can remember to do it. The most important element in bringing about change in the breath is to observe it. Just this alone, conscious attention, often causes the quality of the breath to change on its own, without direction. Keep observing. The following are excellent books that focus on breathing.

Bacci, Ingrid. Effortless Pain Relief. New York: Free Press, 2005.
There is much useful information on relaxed breathing to be found in this outstanding book on releasing pain.

Caponigro, Andy. The Miracle of the Breath. Novato, CA: New World Library, 2005.
Discusses breathing well in order to master fear, heal illness and experience the mystery of life.

Hanh, Thich Nhat. Breathe! You Are Alive: Sutra on the Full Awareness of Breathing. Berkeley: Parallax Press, 1960.
Breathing as a meditative practice. Simple words, profound messages.

Lewis, Dennis. Free Your Breath, Free Your Life. Boston: Shambhala, 2004.
Helpful information and exercises to enhance conscious breathing in order to release stress and increase vitality.

Speads, Carola. Ways to Better Breathing. Rochester, VT: Healing Arts Press, 1992.
This is a classic work on breathing.

Mindfulness/Awareness

Mindfulness is being aware in the present moment by simply paying attention to 'what is.' Mindfulness meditation is a technique that cultivates mindfulness that can then be applied in daily living. We do not have to always sit on a cushion to meditate—we can meditate while washing dishes or driving a car—although the formal practice of meditation can greatly accelerate and enhance our capacity to be mindful. Traditionally, this form of meditation has a spiritual basis in the teachings of the Buddha, with the meditator being on a path to enlightenment and liberation. If this does not work for you, it can be helpful to think of this form of meditation as an art and science of living rather than a religion. In this way, you can focus on the specific benefits to be gained by the practice in order to learn to be more naturally aligned.

It is far easier today to find programs in mindfulness and meditation than it was only a few years ago. Many communities now have opportunities to practice with others locally, and hundreds of hospitals around the country have established mindfulness-based, stress-reduction programs. The following is a very abbreviated listing of many fine books available on the subject and centers that offer retreats and classes.

Gunaratana, Bhante Henepola. Mindfulness: In Plain English. Somerville, MA: Wisdom Publications, 2002.

A classic overview with clear, concise instructions by a man who began as a twelve-year-old monk in Sri Lanka and earned a Ph.D. in philosophy from American University.

Johnson, Will. The Posture of Meditation: A Practical Manual for Meditators of All Traditions. Shambhala: Boston, 1996.

A gem of practical guidance and exercises for working with the posture of meditation, with strategies for integrating these principles into daily life.

Kabat-Zinn, J. Full Catastrophe Living: Using the Wisdom of Your Body and Mind to Face Stress, Pain and Illness. New York: Delacorte, 1990.

One of the first books to address mindfulness and its relationship to stress-reduction and health. A compendium of useful information.

Kabat-Zinn, J. Wherever You Go, There You Are: Mindfulness Meditation in Everyday Life. New York: Hyperion, 1994.

Short, meaningful entries that deepen understanding and appreciation of mindfulness.

Weiss, Andrew. Beginning Mindfulness: Learning the Way of Awareness. Novato, CA: New World Library, 2004.

A practical guide that emphasizes the direct application of mindfulness to daily life.

The following centers offer retreats in mindfulness meditation. They may be able to help you locate programs in your area.

University of Massachusetts Medical School
Center for Mindfulness
55 Lake Avenue North
Worcester, MA 01655
(508) 856-2656
www.umassmed.edu/cfm/mbsr

Insight Meditation Society
1230 Pleasant St.
Barre, MA 01005
(978) 355-4378
www.dharma.org
RC@dharma.org

Shambhala Mountain Center
4921 County Road 68C
Red Feather Lakes, CO 80545
(970) 881-2184
shambhalamountain.org
info@shambhalamountain.org

Spirit Rock Meditation Center
P.O. Box 169
Woodacre, CA 94973
(415) 488-0164
spiritrock.org
info@spiritrock.org

Tathagata Meditation Center
1215 Lucretia Avenue
San Jose, CA
(408) 294-4536
www.tathagata.org

Useful Tools

Sitting Wedge

A foam wedge can help encourage the neutral position of the pelvis when sitting. This is particularly helpful if you do not yet have much of a natural arch at the base of the spine. Wedges also come in handy for anyone who drives a car with a seat that is lower in the back than the front (most cars) that cannot be adjusted to correct this.

There are a variety of wedges on the market in a wide range of prices. Many of these wedges have a cut-out section designed to relieve pressure on the coccyx (tailbone). Although these cushions work, the hole is unnecessary since there is never any pressure on the coccyx when sitting in natural alignment since all contact is with the sit bones. Wedges can be purchased from the sources listed below, among others. After understanding how to sit in natural alignment and doing it successfully, an inflatable ball "chair" can be used comfortably as well.

The Balance Center
560 Oxford Avenue
Palo, Alto, CA 94306
(650) 856-2000
www.balancecenter.com
info@balancecenter.com

Aston Enterprises
(775) 831-8228
www.astonenterprises.com
info@astonenterprises.com
www.sissel-shop-usa.com

In addition to regular foam wedges, this web site also sells an air-filled cushion called Sitfit, which they advertise as combining the buoyancy of sitting on an inflatable ball with the features of a wedge. The good news is that the Sitfit Kinder has been developed for children and is being used in some classrooms to help children sit in a more aligned way.

Please note: None of the above listed products are a substitute for aligned sitting while on a wedge or a ball. Sitting on any surface improperly can force the rib cage to roll backward, straining the back and restricting the diaphragm.

Arch Support for Feet

Arch support can be helpful in keeping your feet in a "scooped" feet position where the weight lands squarely on the heel (Exploration #3) and the leg and ankle muscles are engaged. This is not a substitute for working to strengthen your feet and ankles (see Foot Scoops P. ?) this helps when you are wearing shoes. While there is no way to guarantee that these arch supports will work for you, many people find them helpful. If they don't work, their low price means you are not risking hundreds of dollars for expensive orthotics to find out. For serious foot problems, consult your doctor.

The Balance Center sells quality shoe inserts imported from France. Call (650) 856-2000 or fax (650) 856-0563. You will need to specify shoe size and high or low arch.

Phase 4 Walkfit orthotics has inserts available in three adjustable arch heights. www.walkfit.com

A whole array of products that address a wide range of foot conditions can be found at footsmart.com. There is no guarantee that any of the products here will work for you, although many people have found them helpful.

INDEX

133, 203-204
Balance, ix, xii, xvii, 123-124, 215
bells of alignment, 153, 198
belly, v, xix, 38, 45, 59, 65-66, 68, 75, 77, 90-91, 119, 125, 127, 134-135, 138, 144-145, 147, 155-158, 161, 164-165, 168-169, 174-175, 178-179, 181, 185, 209
bending, vi, xxi, 5, 26, 35, 49, 96, 117-119, 138, 151, 173, 176-178, 189-190, 197-199
biomechanical design, xix, 12, 16-17, 147
Bohr effect feet, 72, 209
bones, xviii-xxi, 3-5, 7-8, 13, 20-22, 24-25, 33-41, 43-47, 49-50, 52-54, 59-64, 66, 69, 74-76, 78-80, 82-83, 85, 87, 91, 93-98, 109-113, 116-117, 119, 125, 127-129, 132, 134, 138, 140, 145, 147, 154-157, 161-162, 164, 166, 168-169, 174, 177-180, 193, 196-199, 205
bracing, 126-127, 161, 177
breathing, v-vi, xx, 4, 6, 12, 34, 37, 42, 59, 65, 70-73, 76, 78, 91, 114-115, 122, 127, 134, 138-139, 144-145, 158, 168-169, 208-209
Buddha, 145, 147, 196, 198
bunions, 84, 87, 194

C
cardiovascular disease, 114, 133, 135
central axis, xix, 8, 20, 23, 28, 37-41, 43-45, 49, 53-54, 61-63, 69, 101, 123-124, 141-146, 152, 204
cervical spine, 141
children v, x, xix, 17, 28, 35, 51, 71, 104, 109, 205
    computers and, 108

feet and, 80, 84, 167
loss of alignment and, 97-99, 125, 146
natural alignment and, 20-21, 95-96, 98, 118-119
sports and, 106-107

chimpanzees, 51, 206
chiropractic, 7, 123
chronic hyperventilation syndrome, 72, 134
clavicle, 50, 191
compression, 34-37, 68, 111, 116, 128-130, 134, 141
Couch, Jean, vii, ix, xii, xvii, xxi, 123-124, 187, 195, 197
cultural conditioning, xviii, 9, 14, 151
culture, xiv, xix, 3, 8, 14, 16, 21, 47, 52, 144-145

D
diaphragm, 4-5, 71-74, 78, 90-91, 114, 134, 168, 207
Durkheim, Karlfried Graf, 144

E
evolution, 81, 204
evolutionary design, 36, 38
exhalation, 70-71, 73, 193

F
fight or flight response, 59, 134
fitness , xi-xii, xviii, 3, 6-8, 12, 14, 19, 26, 40, 45, 75, 111-112, 114-115, 145, 197
flexibility, xiv, 12, 19, 23, 26, 33, 81, 86, 113, 116-117
foot scoops, vi, 166-167, 199
force/counterforce, vii, 34-35, 48, 69-70,